THE PLEASURE CENTER

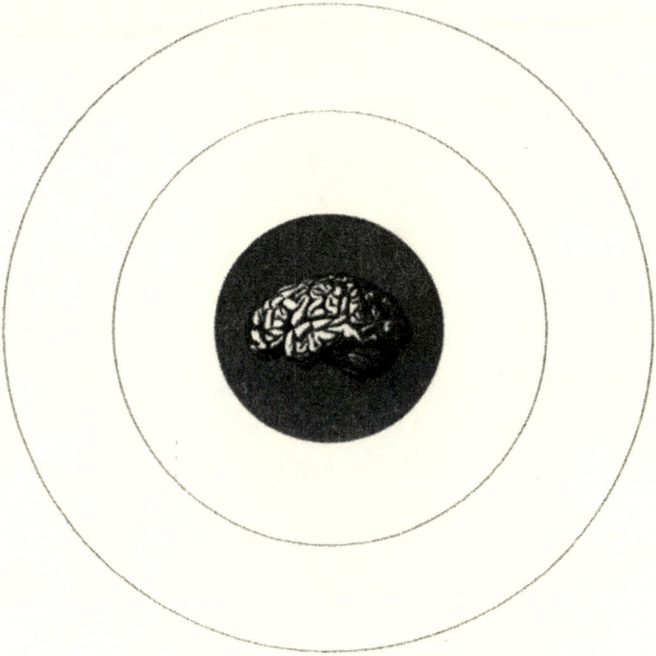

OXFORD UNIVERSITY PRESS NEW YORK 2009

THE PLEASURE CENTER

TRUST YOUR ANIMAL INSTINCTS

MORTEN L. KRINGELBACH

Oxford University Press

Oxford University Press, Inc., publishes works that further
Oxford University's objective of excellence
in research, scholarship, and education.

Oxford New York
Auckland Cape Town Dar es Salaam Hong Kong Karachi
Kuala Lumpur Madrid Melbourne Mexico City Nairobi
New Delhi Shanghai Taipei Toronto

With offices in
Argentina Austria Brazil Chile Czech Republic France Greece
Guatemala Hungary Italy Japan Poland Portugal Singapore
South Korea Switzerland Thailand Turkey Ukraine Vietnam

Published by Oxford University Press, Inc.
198 Madison Avenue, New York, New York 10016
www.oup.com

Library of Congress Cataloging-in-Publication Data

Kringelbach, Morten L.

The pleasure center : trust your animal instincts
/ Morten L. Kringelbach.
p. cm.
Includes bibliographical references (p.) and index.
ISBN 978-0-19-532285-9
1. Pleasure. 2. Desire. I. Title.
BF515.K5813 2008
152.4'2—dc22
2008023787

3 5 7 9 8 6 4 2

Printed in the United States of America
on acid-free paper

PREFACE

Few would choose to live a life without emotions, yet at the same time many people believe that our emotions are obstacles to intelligent action. Emotion is not reason's antithesis. On the contrary, it is fighting the pleasures and desires of life that is irrational, because they are essential to all human behavior. This book will help you understand the underpinnings of emotion in your brain. Pleasure (and its corollary, avoidance of pain) is central to this understanding, as it is the currency for all of our decisions, actions, and experiences. A better understanding of how pleasure and desire work in our brains can lead to important insights about our nature and, in time, may also improve treatment for those whose depression or mental illness robs them of their pleasure.

I investigate the many facets of pleasure, desire and emotion by probing the reward systems of the brain and, along the way, uncover the spectrum of human experience from the sensory inputs and memory, via emotion, through learning, decisions and consciousness, to madness, drugs and sex. I also present some of the most interesting new scientific discoveries about pleasure and desire. Understanding and accepting how pleasures and desires arise in the complex interaction between the brain's activity and our subjective experiences can help us to make better decisions, find what helps us enjoy life, and lead happier lives.

CONTENTS

THE PLEASURE CENTER

1

THE CHALLENGE

Know Thyself?

> The knowledge of good and evil is nothing else but the emotions of pleasure or pain, in so far as we are conscious thereof.
>
> Baruch Spinoza (1632–1677)

"Know thyself" was inscribed on the portico of the temple at Delphi, and the apparent uncanny accuracy of the oracular utterances depended precisely on that self-understanding. Nothing has interested us more than understanding ourselves—and other people. After thousands of years of searching, we are finally coming closer to a better understanding of the brain. More refined insights into its functions were not possible until the recent invention of new brain scanning techniques that have allowed us to track brain activity. Similarly further insights have come from deep-brain stimulation techniques that have allowed us to help patients with otherwise treatment-resistant disorders.

CHALLENGING BRAINS

These new discoveries in brain science—or *neuroscience*, as it is also known—give us new insights into the human brain and the basis for a better understanding of ourselves. Indeed, research into pleasures, desires, and emotions may well force us to reconsider some of our basic and cherished beliefs. Pleasure is so important to our actions because it is central to how our brains are guided and sculpted through learning. From early childhood, the self is created in the brain through a struggle between genetics and flexible learning. Human brains are not blank slates on which anything can be written. Rather, the brain's fundamental structure has already been determined by genetic material assembled during our evolutionary history, and so certain universal forms of learning take place as part of the potential that is always present in nature. Language is a good example of a potential that is universal, or shared by all human beings. These universal learning potentials form the foundation of all our abilities. Although human experience—and thus our learning potential—is limited, it is flexible, so the self may take certain forms that can be divided into broad categories, which we call personality types.

THE ANATOMY OF PLEASURE

Pleasure and pain are essential to desires, motivations, and emotions. Experience makes it clear that we will always try to obtain that which gives us pleasure and avoid that which does not. Our subjective experience of pleasure is rather extraordinary. Pleasure appears to evaporate when we direct our attention to it. The more we focus on the pleasure itself, the more it slips away. Yet, this is not the case when we direct our attention to the events leading to pleasure. The experience of pleasure involves intentionality and at least four distinct stages: engagement, acceptance, continuation, and subsequent return. For example, the pleasure of chocolate involves choosing chocolate over other foods, eating the first bite, and continuing the pleasant experience of eating until full. In the future, we will eat more chocolate. The scenario is similar in situations where we encounter someone we desire: We choose a person to stop and engage with; decide whether they actually are interesting (and interested in us); try to make the conversation last as long as possible; and desire to return as soon as possible.

We generally experience pleasure and pain in one of the three combinations: pleasant–unpleasant, relaxed–tense, or quiet–excited. The perceived pleasantness or unpleasantness is not usually experienced entirely in our selves, but rather depends on the perceived object or experience. How we anticipate and evaluate the object or experience are core aspects of pleasure and pain. Pleasure and pain are linked to reward values that guide how we learn, our preferences, and our behavioral priorities. This type of hedonic evaluation was named "utility" by the English philosopher Jeremy Bentham, following the Greek philosopher Epicurus. Although philosophers have remained skeptical of all versions of utility theory, many neuroscientists and economists have come to believe that the anticipatory and evaluative elements of pleasure are fundamental to decision making. One example is the recent Nobel laureate in Economics, Daniel Kahneman, who reintroduced the concept of utility to describe how pleasure can help optimize decision making. Kahneman also created some important distinctions in his description of utility. He distinguishes between *experience utility* and *decision utility.* Experience utility is how much we like or dislike a choice we are making. Decision utility relates to whether we want or don't want the object of the choice.

Neuroscientists now study the more subjective nature of pleasure by matching people's reports of how much they are enjoying an experience with scans of their brain activity during the experience. Animals can't describe in words how much they are enjoying a particular experience, but the pioneering research of the American neuroscientist Kent Berridge has shown that pleasure often entails species-specific hedonic behaviors. For example, rats and mice contently lick their lips when given sweet-tasting food, whereas bad-tasting food will lead them to gape, shake their heads, and frantically wipe their mouths—just as infants do. By measuring the frequency of these behaviors, Berridge got a good measure of the rats' hedonic experience, which he then linked with measurements of their brain activity. As we shall see later, Berridge has shown that pleasure has at least two subcomponents, liking and wanting, which use partly separate brain pathways and may correspond to Kahneman's distinction between experience utility and decision utility.

Pleasure is produced by the activity and interaction of many different brain regions. Some of the processing is conscious, but much—if not most—of this hedonic processing proceeds nonconsciously, so that we have rather little conscious insight into these processes. Studying them may give rise to a better understanding of our emotional brain. It may also force us to reconsider our beliefs about rationality and free will because if we are aware of only a small fraction of what goes on in our brain, how many of our decisions are we really consciously making? How reliable is our memory? How rational are our actions?

PLEASURE AND PAIN IN THE BRAIN

Pleasure and pain are closely linked with each other, but opinions differ over whether they are opposites or just different aspects of the same thing. While a stimulus rarely makes us both approach and avoid it at the same time, it is nevertheless clear that one can feel both pleasure and displeasure. These experiences and memories, as when we laugh at a happy memory but miss those involved or long for the return of past pleasures, are often described as bittersweet.

Desire is situated at the interface between motivation, pleasure, and reward. Most standard definitions relate desire to motivation, in the sense that if we desire something, we are motivated to bring it about. The Portuguese philosopher Baruch Spinoza wrote that "pleasure is the transition of a man from a less to a greater perfection," where perfection is the extent to which that man has realized his desires. The Canadian philosopher Timothy Schroeder has argued against such standard accounts of desire, instead linking intrinsic desire directly with the reward systems of the brain.

REASONABLE FEELINGS?

Recent research has shown that humans are mainly emotional beings who only occasionally use reason to their advantage. This insight contrasts sharply with the commonly held belief that human behavior can be explained through reason and rationality. Human history, however, also contrasts sharply with this belief by demonstrating that rationality has usually failed to rule, or to even affect, human behavior. Despite the fact that people can rationalize the motives for their actions after the fact, and identify the "best" option in a given situation, there is now mounting evidence that these subsequent rationalizations have little influence on the decision to take the action in the first place. What has been missing in how we see ourselves is an understanding of those desires, pleasures, emotions, and feelings that are central to our lives. Throughout history, emotion and rationality have been seen as opposing forces, with emotion being regarded as a lower animal instinct because it was out of the reach of reason, and therefore best suppressed. If we develop a proper understanding of our emotions, we will see that they do not conflict with reason.

THE BRAIN CAROUSEL

Fighting desires that we don't understand is both irrational and a huge waste of energy and resources. We are not suggesting giving in to all of one's impulses. Some, yes. But others we quite rightly need to resist. However, without understanding them, we will not know how to resist them.

Pleasure and desire underlie all of our decisions, so if we understand, accept, and even listen to them, we will not only be able to save time and energy, but we will—believe it or not—gain wisdom. Our emotions and desires are one of the only tools we have for understanding ourselves and others. Our emotions and desires have evolved over thousands of years because developing this type of an understanding is one of the best ways to protect ourselves and improve our lives. To understand our emotions and desires, we have to know how their components work in our mind and body. To that end, each chapter in this book explains a different component.

Chapter 2 shows how pleasure and reward values underlie our decisions.

Chapter 3 tries to grapple with our subjective conscious experience of pleasure.

Chapter 4 explores how difficult it has been to understand emotions by exploring how scientists have struggled to quantify them and their links to pleasure and desire.

Chapter 5 investigates the basis of our sensory experiences. Understanding these experiences will give us a basis for understanding our sensory pleasures, which are the likely building blocks and templates for the rest of our higher-order pleasures.

Chapter 6 investigates memory systems in the brain and their role in memories of pleasure.

Chapter 7 investigates learning in the brain, and how pleasure plays an important if undervalued role in education.

Chapter 8 focuses on the lack of pleasure in depression and mental illness.

Chapte 9 describes the effects of stimulants that can cause addiction, which can be thought of as wanting without liking.

Chapter 10 uncovers some of the pleasures of sex, from desire to climax.

Chapter 11 concludes the book by looking forward to what we can do with these ideas to improve both our individual lives and the world as a whole.

Brief Definition of Pleasure

Pleasure can be defined as a way of fulfilling the evolutionary imperatives of survival and procreation. This leads to a classification of pleasure in *fundamental* (sensory, sexual, and social pleasures) and *higher-order pleasures* (for example, monetary, artistic, musical, altruistic, and transcendent pleasures).

Pleasure is not a sensation but is instead linked to the anticipation and subsequent evaluation of stimuli. Pleasure is thus a complex psychological phenomenon with close links to the reward systems of the brain and as such consists of both conscious and nonconscious processes. There are at least three fundamental elements to pleasure: wanting, liking, and learning. The brain regions and brain mechanisms of these subcomponents of pleasure can be studied in both humans and other animals.

2

DECISIONS

Social Intelligence in the World

Those who will not reason, Perish in the act;
Those who will not act, Perish for that reason.

W.H. Auden (1907–1973)

A 3-year-old boy climbed the fence surrounding the enclosure for the great apes in the Chicago zoo and fell some 20 feet onto the concrete below, rendering him unconscious. The lowland gorilla Binti Jua picked up the boy and sat gently cradling him for a while. She then carried him back to an entrance to the enclosure and continued walking with her 17-month-old baby on her back, as if nothing had happened. The boy eventually recovered fully.

Binti Jua quickly became a minor celebrity, and some politicians used her actions as an example of the altruism needed in society. If such moral behavior can be exhibited by a gorilla, then why is it so difficult to find in humans? However, some scientists argued that Binti Jua learned this behavior from humans in the first place, as she had been raised by humans and had used a doll to practice her maternal skills. For them, Binti Jua's behavior was not a moral act, but solely a symptom of confused maternal instinct. Arguments about confused maternal instincts seem weak when you consider that Binti's maternal needs were fulfilled—she carried her own baby on her back throughout the incident. It is also difficult to see how a highly intelligent animal, such as a gorilla, would be unable to distinguish a fully clothed boy from her own gorilla baby. There is some research to support the claims of morality over confusion. The Dutch primatologist Frans de Waal and other scientists have claimed that the higher primates display at least basic moral behavior. If higher primates can be said to be capable of acting morally, it may well be the end of the long-cherished notion that humans are the sole moral animals. Whatever its cause, it seems difficult to argue against Binti Jua's act being positive and intelligent, and being what she wanted to do, what pleased her. In fact, a growing body of research suggests that feelings of pleasure play a key role in both our conscious decisions and how we understand our nonconscious ones.

Although pleasure and desire underlie all of our decisions, this does not mean that we are driven solely by self-interest. Some of our greatest pleasures in life come from social interactions with others. We are very social animals, and we share this sociality with other types of animals. If we are to understand our emotional brain, we have to understand what drives our social brain. We can mirror ourselves in the other higher primates and see that despite our cultural veneer, we are still, for better or worse, similar to other animals, particularly in our social behavior. It is well documented that chimpanzees show regionally determined behavior that probably should be deemed as at least the beginnings of culture. Many of the moral qualities we appreciate—and detest—in other humans are found in other primates. Humans also have animal vices that we keep on a short leash.

THROUGH THE LOOKING GLASS

We use each other as social mirrors. This behavior begins early—newborn babies appear to imitate *others'* facial expressions to relate their *own* feelings. Of course, as blind children exhibit normal facial expressions, there must be a large degree of genetic influence as well. Experiments with primates have shown *mirror neurons* in the frontal part of the brain. These are neurons that act both when an animal itself reaches for an object, and when it observes another animal reaching for an object. The discovery of mirror neurons demonstrated that monkeys have mental representations of the actions of others, which are important for understanding the intentions of others. In humans, this ability has developed so far that we continuously try to read other peoples' intentions on their faces.

In 1970, the American psychologist Gordon Gallup carried out an experiment in which he placed a dot on the forehead of a chimpanzee, so that it could only be seen when the chimp looked in a mirror. Gallup's experiment showed that most animals are unable to recognize themselves in a mirror. Chimpanzees, bonobos, orangutans, and dolphins—but not, for example, gorillas—will notice the dot. This self-recognition also becomes easier with age: chimpanzees appear to recognize themselves at around 6 years; human infants exhibit self-recognition at around 1½ years. As passing the mirror test is age dependent, it is possible that a hierarchy exists in the brain for the acquisition of advanced mental abilities. An individual must always acquire the capability of self-recognition before acquiring the ability to attribute intentional motives, desires, and goals to others.

The Beginning of Morality

Gallup's discovery of self-recognition in chimpanzees was the first step in showing whether they have the prerequisites for morality, such as intentional behavior, desires, pleasures, and emotions. More recent experiments have investigated the ability of chimpanzees to see themselves and others as thinking beings. One important experiment tried to verify whether a chimpanzee can use intentional knowledge to determine where food has been hidden. Initially, a researcher hid food in one of the four boxes while another researcher would wear a bag over his head or leave the room, so it was clear that only one of the researchers knew the location of the food. This researcher always would point to the correct box, but the other researcher would point at random. Using only the information from the first researcher, the chimpanzee would find the food, demonstrating that it was able to use intentional knowledge.

Morality may have developed as a result of the social mirror found in gregarious animals. Each individual is constantly being monitored by others. The resulting interplay produces the elements that constitute morality: sympathy, attachment, helping, emotional bonds, and presiding social rules. Further attributes include adaptation and special care for the injured and handicapped. Also important is reciprocity, such as the abilities to give, act, and avenge, including aggression toward rule-breakers. These, in turn, require the ability to handle conflicts through mediation and the constant maintenance of stable social relations. All of these characteristics are well documented in a number of social animals, but they are far more developed in humans, which is probably among the reasons that some people think that humans are the only moral animals. It might be worth remembering that, as with so much in nature, the question of morality is probably more one of degree rather than of kind.

Cute Infants

At the heart of morality lies the very special social bond between parents and infants. Charles Darwin and the Nobel Prize–winning zoologist Konrad Lorenz proposed that infantile facial features are central to this bond. Lorenz argued that infantile features serve as "innate releasing mechanisms" for affection and nurturing in adult humans and that most of the features are evident in the face, including a relatively large head, predominance of the brain capsule, large and low-lying eyes, and bulging cheeks. These features increase the infant's chance of survival by evoking parental responses.

My research team also found a key difference in the early brain activity of normal adults (who are not parents) when they viewed infant faces as compared to when they viewed adult faces. Only infant faces elicited early activity in the medial orbitofrontal cortex, which has previously been implicated in reward-related behavior. We found that the processing of both adult and infant faces elicits a wave of brain activity starting in visual cortices and spreading along ventral and dorsal pathways. However, at around 130 ms after seeing an infant face, activity was found in the medial orbitofrontal cortex (Figure 2.1). The medial orbitofrontal cortex is a key region of the emotional brain and appears to be related to the ongoing monitoring of salient reward-related stimuli in the environment. The medial orbitofrontal

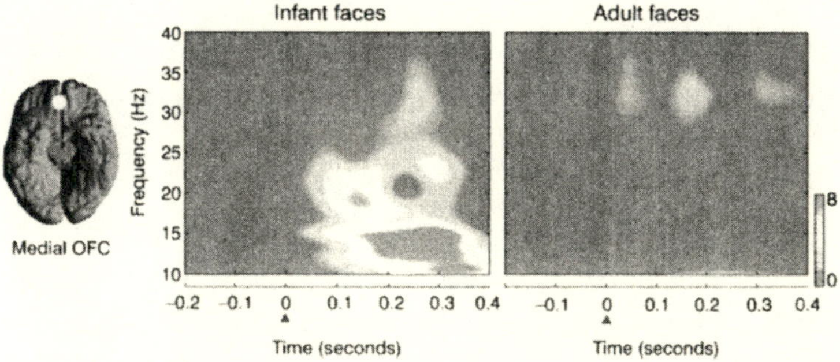

Figure 2.1 The pleasure of infant faces. Normal adults watched infant and adult faces while we measured the activity in their brains. The infant faces evoked early activity in the medial orbitofrontal cortex (left and middle panel), which was not the case when they saw the adult faces (right panel). This marker for parental instinct could potentially help identify those parents who are likely to suffer from postnatal depression.

cortex may provide the necessary emotional tagging of infant faces that predisposes us to treat infant faces as special, and so play a key role in establishing the parental bond. We also have a disproportionate interest in the infants of other animal species. It is likely that apes share similar brain mechanisms, which probably also contributed to Binti Jua's behavior toward the human child.

INTELLIGENT ACTIONS

What is intelligence quotient (IQ)? The IQ test began in 1904, in a test battery invented by French researchers, Alfred Binet and Theodor Simon. They were asked by the government to find a method for identifying children of lesser ability so those children could get help to improve. Their psychometric tests spread quickly. A *quotient* was invented as the ratio of real and mental age, and normality was defined as *100*. According to definition, 50% of all children will score between 90 and 110, precocious children will score higher, and so-called retarded children, much lower. Because this quotient was quickly seen as a measure of human intelligence, it became known as *Intelligence Quotient*, or IQ. But is it really meaningful to use a single number to denote the capacity and potential of an individual? These measures are useful to the extent that they capture something essential, but are still limited. Few people now claim that an IQ score is more than just one of many indicators for mental abilities, and some researchers have suggested that other measures are far more meaningful. Creativity and emotional intelligence are the most popular suggestions.

Mildly Retarded Analyses

Recent studies have shown that the environment plays a much larger role in IQ than most hardboiled geneticists have been willing to admit. For children of all races, IQ increases with education. The French psychologist Michel Duyme and his colleagues followed a large group of adopted children over three decades. When the children were adopted between the ages of four and six, each had an IQ below 86, which is defined as *mildly retarded*. In many cases, these children had been abused and neglected during their infancy. By the time the children entered puberty, each child's IQ had adapted to that of their adopted family. Before this study, it was widely believed that the influence of the environment had to take place within the first 6 years of life. The study showed that the possibility for children to improve their IQ score depends strongly on the environment into which they are adopted.

This study is one of many that have undermined the conclusions from Herrnstein and Murray's biased and racist book, *The Bell Curve*, which sold, sadly, over half a million copies. Since the publication of this book, other researchers have had the opportunity to reanalyze its data. The result is that many of the conclusions in the book appear to be just plain wrong. Notably, Herrnstein and Murray proposed that the genetic influence on intelligence is at least 60% and probably closer to 80%. Much other research has shown that the number is probably in the area of 50%, and may be even lower. The rest is determined by environmental factors such as social environment, diet, and education. On the basis of these studies, it is tempting to ask whether IQ tests are more culturally biased than previously acknowledged. Probably the best thing to be said for the *The Bell Curve* is that it sparked interest in the continued debate on the importance of intelligence in the organization of society. It is increasingly clear that IQ tests are not particularly good tools for creating a better society. IQ tests primarily reveal many things about the people who created them, but only a tiny and perhaps even obscure fraction of what goes on in our brains. These limitations do not mean that IQ tests are useless, but that they must be supplemented with other measures, and regarded with a healthy dose of skepticism.

Intelligence in the Brain

What is the relationship between IQ and intelligence? The answer depends on how intelligence is defined, and the definition must be based on what we know about brain function, as the brain forms the basis of our intelligence. To get closer to an answer, we need to understand how the smallest parts of the brain function in neural networks that underlie all of our thoughts, emotions, and actions. This may in turn help us to better understand what might be the machinery of intelligent actions.

The brain is far too often compared with the computer, but there are a couple of important things we can learn from this comparison. Brains are patched together from various components that have evolved over time, whereas computers are designed and constructed from logical principles. The differences in design and history mean that brains, like computers, are good at some things and not as good at others. For example, the human brain is relatively good at surviving, reproducing, and making decisions in very complex environments, but it is not as good at making exact calculations, which are seldom needed for survival. By contrast, computers do not need to survive or reproduce, and are rarely asked to make their own decisions, yet they can do endless calculations.

A neuron is one of the smallest, but most significant, parts of the brain. Neurons are small, advanced machines that can summate activity from each other and decide whether this activity should be transferred to yet other neurons. We are still learning about the functioning of neurons. Neuron connections create the neural networks that form the biological basis of brain activity. A collection of neurons can initiate cascades of activity from one neuron to the next, just like dominos falling onto each other. But unlike dominos, neurons will continue to repeat this activity and can decide if and when they will contact the next part of the chain. The central property of neurons is that they are able to learn. A neuron can selectively change its influence on other neurons, which would be like dominos deciding which of the other dominos would get the biggest push. In the central nervous system, there are many different types of neurons in many different shapes and with many different functions. For instance, clear anatomical differences are found between the neurons that receive sensory information from the skin and those in the main motor cortex that control motor movements.

More important than the function of a single neuron are the possibilities for learning that are endowed by networks of neurons. This learning forms the basis for our mental abilities and intelligence. In 1948, Canadian psychologist Donald Hebb proposed the fundamental principle for learning in neural networks: that synapses can change their strength so that they can influence other neurons more or less. A more complete description of what we have learned about neural networks in the brain from using computers is described in readable details elsewhere. Here we are concerned with understanding the mechanisms that underlie the decisions made by our brain all the time. For this purpose, the study of artificial neural networks has contributed quite a lot to our understanding.

THE SOCIAL CHOICES OF THE BRAIN

We are now in a much better position to assess how the real neural networks in the brain make decisions. One of the hallmarks of human nature in general and social intelligence in particular is our flexible behavior. A fundamental characteristic of social intelligence is the ability to quickly change our behavior. Our flexible social skills are already being honed as children and young adolescents, when we quickly become very adept at forming and breaking alliances within and between groups, and we engage in complex social interactions. This type of social intelligence, untested by conventional intelligence tests, is crucial for social behavior. It must be a major reason for our relative evolutionary success and probably is better than IQ at predicting how well a person will do in life.

Although it is obviously important that we can learn arbitrary associations between stimuli, it is equally important that we can relatively easily break these associations and relearn others. If we learn that choosing a certain stimulus leads to a reward, it would be maladaptive to keep choosing the stimulus when it is no longer associated with a reward, but instead with, say, a punishment. We need to be able to adapt or reverse the learning patterns when things change. This kind of learning is called *reversal learning* in the psychological literature. The English psychologist Susan Iversen and American neurophysiologist Mortimer Mishkin showed that when the inferior prefrontal convexity and parts of the lateral orbitofrontal cortex were damaged in monkeys, they became significantly impaired in object reversal learning. This elegant and very significant result has had a huge influence over subsequent research.

BRAIN SCANNERS AND EMOTIONAL DAMAGE

Subsequent experiments with monkeys and humans have confirmed Iversen and Mishkin's results. In particular, it has been shown that lesions to the orbitofrontal cortex lead to changes in social behavior. Emotional and social problems following brain damage can, however, be subtle and may remain undiagnosed with psychological tests, which creates its own problems for the family that has to live with the often-radical changes in personality.

The Canadian neurologist Antoine Bechara and his colleagues created a gambling task to detect the subtle cognitive deficits in brain-damaged patients who are unable to change their behavior when choosing between card decks with associated monetary gains and losses. Even if the patients were aware that it would be better to choose the deck with small wins and small losses than the deck with the big wins and even bigger losses, they continued to choose the deck with the big wins. These patients had lesions in the orbitofrontal cortex and other brain structures, including the amygdala.

Our research group developed a similar gambling task. The subjects' task was to determine by trial and error which of two stimuli is the more profitable choice, to keep track of it, and reverse their choice when a reversal occurred in the stimuli. We designed the task so that the actual reversal event was difficult to determine because money can be won or lost on both stimuli. In general, the choice of the rewarding stimulus would give larger rewards and smaller punishments. The converse was true of the punishing stimulus, in that losing a large amount of money would often signal that a reversal had occurred. Patients with circumscribed bilateral lesions of the lateral part of the orbitofrontal cortex have great difficulties in continuing to win at this gambling task. However, in contrast to the Bechara gambling task, our task is well suited for use with neuroimaging, so we can use it to find out how the brain keeps track of wins and losses.

Scanning a group of normal participants, we showed that they use the orbitofrontal cortex to keep track of the rewarding stimuli. But we found a dissociation between the medial and the lateral parts of the orbitofrontal cortex, where one part was correlated with the amount of wins, and the other was correlated with the amount of losses. In contrast to previous experiments in both humans and other primates, we used money, which is one of the most abstract kinds of stimuli used for reward and punishment. This finding gave us our first insight into how our brains keep track of wins and losses of even abstract stimuli, revealing important characteristics of our emotional brain.

SOCIAL FACE EXPRESSIONS

To understand social behavior, we designed a task that uses faces as the primary stimuli, which gave us the opportunity to investigate some of the fundamental attributes of simple social relationships. The overall goal is to keep track of the mood of two people presented together. Although they begin with neutral facial expressions, one person smiles when the subjects select an image of a "happy" person, and the other frowns when the subject selects an image of an "angry" person. The object of the task is to continue to select the "happy" person and receive smiles in return. But suddenly the "happy" person will become angry, while the other person will become "happy." Now the subject has to learn to select the image of the other person and not select the image of the previously happy person. To control for the possibility that the changes might be linked to only those brain regions involved in processing angry facial expressions, the participants were also asked to perform a task where the angry person remained neutral as a sign that a behavioral change was needed. This work gave us a precise understanding of which parts of the brain are linked to changing social behavior. It turns out that this task elicits significant brain activity in the frontal part of the brain and specifically in the lateral orbitofrontal and anterior cingulate cortices.

CONSCIOUS FREE WILL?

All kinds of choices require weighing the potential reward and punishment. In the best cases, this weighing may lead to good rational decisions. Many people feel that their consciousness is a key player in such free rational choices that control most, if not all, of their lives. But it is also possible that this intuition, like so much of our conscious self-insight, is an illusion.

Let us look briefly at rationality. Making a truly completely rational decision is difficult because it would require gathering all the possible information needed to make the best decision. But there is never enough time to gather that much information, and even if there were, it would be next to impossible to know whether it all had been gathered. Psychological research has shown that, in stark contrast to trying to gather even most of the relevant information, people rarely take much notice at all of the available information. Evolution has configured our brains such that even when we are not under the influence of drugs, fatigue, or strong emotions, our decisions are often deeply irrational. There are many examples of the collapse of rationality in our everyday behavior, such as that people might travel a long distance to save $5 on an object that would cost $10 in a nearby shop, but it's less likely that they would go out of their way to save $5 on a $10,000 object, even though it is the same amount saved in both cases.

But do we act in these ways as a consequence of *conscious* reason? We know that patients with brain damage are unable to do what they say they should. Even more of a concern is the scientific data concluding that we are making up the reasons for our actions as we go along. Although we may be able to rationalize most of our decisions, these rationalizations do not necessarily reflect what happened when we made the decisions. One interpretation of this data is that actions spring from nonconscious processing that is only consciously interpreted after the fact.

The neurophysiologists Hans Helmut Kornhuber and Lüder Deecke showed that neural activity occurs up to 2 seconds before we do something as simple as moving a finger. This activity is known as *readiness potential*. The American neurophysiologist Benjamin Libet tried to extend these experiments to get at the timing of decisions. He asked human participants to move their finger whenever they felt like it, and also to report the position of their hand when they felt the urge to move their finger. This urge typically occurs around half a second before the movement, but *after* the neural activity related to the readiness potential. In other words, brain activity related to the finger movement seems to occur a half or a whole second before we become aware of it.

This conclusion could be taken to mean that our free will emerges from what is essentially nonconscious processing, which has led some researchers to propose that free will does not exist. But this is not the only possible explanation of the data. If one accepts that we have only limited insight into a small fraction of our brain processes, it follows that our decisions can in fact remain free even without the involvement of consciousness. Such an interpretation could be taken to mean that although *conscious* free will might be an illusion, *nonconscious* free will is likely. There are of course more radical interpretations: the definition of consciousness is flawed;

the conscious/nonconscious dichotomy is a misleading way of framing the discussion; conscious and nonconscious are endpoints of a spectrum of brain activity that contains intermediate points as well. The main point is clear, however, namely that nonconscious brain processing are likely to play a greater part in our actions than we think and may play a central role in the construction of the self.

The preferences and intuitions that emerge through emotional learning are fundamental. We constantly associate behavior with reward and punishment, which have a goal of maximizing pleasure. The use of nonconscious brain processing might be helpful in that it creates the possibility of avoiding bottlenecks in decision making. Conscious brain processing is serial and slow, and rarely can process more than nine elements at a time. Nonconscious brain processing can manipulate much larger amounts of information, which means that our decisions can be influenced by information from the senses that are not normally consciously available.

An example of the power of subliminal stimuli to influence our conscious decisions comes from the research of the American neuroscientist Kent Berridge. Human participants were shown images of neutral faces and asked to determine the gender of each face. At the end of the experiment, participants were asked to pour as much juice as they wanted into a glass and drink it. The participants were pleased by this because they had been asked to refrain from drinking before the experiment. Just before presentation of each neutral face, another face had been presented very briefly. The presentation was so quick that none of the participants noticed, yet the facial expression had influenced their subsequent behavior. When an angry face was subliminally presented, participants on average poured and drank significantly less than when they were shown a happy face. In a related experiment, participants also would not pay as much for the same drink when subliminally shown angry faces as they would when subliminally shown happy faces.

Our feeling of conscious free will is paradoxical in the sense that it is hard to see how it can arise in our biological brains. At the same time, we clearly need to feel that we are in control of our actions. It remains a possibility that our conscious self could be nothing more than a passenger with highly developed skills for post hoc rationalizations of our actions. Because pleasure is a key part of our post hoc conscious appraisal, it could be that the ability and need to feel pleasure are among the driving forces of consciousness. Beneath the pleasures and feelings of our conscious lives lurk emotions that are constant undercurrents of extensive nonconscious brain processing. They are important because they provide the drive to sustain life, to reproduce, and thus to remain in motion. This nonconscious brain processing is not the same as the subconscious described by Sigmund Freud. Most of these brain processes are not repressed, as he presumed, but rather nonconscious in the sense that they are part of brain activity that we can never gain conscious access to.

Much of our pleasure comes from social interactions; we're learning more about how they originate in the brain and the role of emotions in them. The word "emotion," is derived from Latin, and means that which "moves us to action." It is this incentive for action that makes emotions adaptive from an evolutionary perspective. It is also the reason that it always feels like something to be conscious. We may be well advised to trust some of our emotional intuitions in shaping adaptive decisions.

● ● ● HAPPINESS LESSONS

Social skills should not be underrated, and could arguably be counted as a type of intelligence.

Don't be too slow to adapt to changing conditions. Understand that what is rewarding at one point in time may not continue to be rewarding (in fact, may turn costly) at a different time.

FURTHER READING

Humans are not the only animals to make decisions, so understanding the decisions of other greater apes could be important. I recommend the following books: de Waal, F. B. M. (1994). *Good Natured: Origins of Right and Wrong in Humans and Other Animals.* Cambridge, Mass: Harvard University Press.

Wrangham, R. W., McGrew, W. C., de Waal, F. B. M. & Heltne, P. (1994). *Chimpanzee Cultures.* Cambridge, Mass: Harvard University Press.

Our decisions draw upon the neural networks in the brain. For those interested in neural networks, I recommend the following book: Cotterill, R. M. J. (1998). *Enchanted Looms. Conscious Networks in Brains and Computers.* Cambridge: Cambridge University Press.

I also strongly recommend the following antidote to rabid rationality: Sutherland, S. (1992). *Irrationality. The Enemy within.* London: Constable and Co.

3

CONSCIOUSNESS

Artificial Pleasures and Desires in Other Bodies?

We shall not cease from exploration
And the end of all our exploring
Will be to arrive where we started
And know the place for the first time.

T.S. Eliot (1888–1965)

When John Steinbeck described consciousness as a tragic miracle, he meant that although our sophisticated understanding and awareness of what is happening in the present and what is likely to happen in the future gives us the freedom to make choices and follow our desires, we also know that we will not live forever. That is, we are all aware, on some level, that we are living a tragedy, in that sooner or later we will have to leave everything that gives meaning to our lives. In the face of this reality, however, most of us remain full of optimism, continuing to form and nurture the relationships and interests that create the tragedy.

Our subjective experience is perhaps *the* defining characteristic of consciousness. As we have seen, several brain regions are possible candidates for mediating this experience. The orbitofrontal cortex, anterior cingulate cortex, insular cortex, and ventral striatum have been clearly implicated in the hedonic networks that contribute to shaping our behavior and our subjective experience.

Our survival depends on access to food, and our senses of taste and smell are among the building blocks of the brain's reward systems—the same systems that fuel our interest in sex and drugs. Even for omnivorous animals such as humans, it can be difficult to maintain stable food intake in different, often hostile, climates. Our so-called higher cognitive abilities have developed through evolution to support the necessary cognitive skills underlying advanced food gathering. The study of food intake could be the central tool in understanding human nature, particularly as it can give us precise information about the neural correlates of pleasure and aversion.

STATES OF CONSCIOUSNESS

Sleep is a strange state of consciousness in which we spend a significant portion of our lives. It is also a complex entity that can shed light on our other conscious states. Scientists, however, don't know much about it. In fact, it was only during the beginning of the last century that they began to be able to say something a bit more meaningful about sleep than resurrecting some version of the ancient Greek idea that it is a short death. Sleeping quite often involves dreams, which have always been treated with the utmost respect. The time spent "in the arms of Morpheus," however, was always regarded as wasted until neuroscience research showed that sleep is as important to us as breathing.

The scientific study of sleep began with the discovery that it is possible to measure brain activity. What scientists measure are tiny electrical charges from the billions of neurons in the brain. Measurements are taken on the outside of the skull using a technique called *electroencephalography* (EEG). Although this activity is constantly changing, it follows a certain pattern during sleep, always moving through four phases. REM sleep, the fourth and most renowned phase, was discovered in 1953. It is called *REM* for the rapid eye movements that occur while the rest of the body remains paralyzed (or almost paralyzed, as men often have an erection during this phase). Before birth, babies spend almost half of their sleeping time in REM sleep, but as we get older, we need both less sleep and less REM. If people are awakened during the REM phase, they are highly likely to report having had a complex dream. Although we may dream during the other three phases, our recollection of these dreams is often limited to a single thought or mental image, rather than having the narrative quality of our dreams during REM sleep.

DO OTHER ANIMALS DREAM?

Nearly all mammals dream and even birds show signs of dreaming as hatchlings. In other animals, REM sleep is called *paradoxical sleep*. Paradoxical sleep is thought to have entered evolutionary history approximately 180 million years ago, and must carry quite important advantages given that the presence of predators makes it potentially dangerous to become paralyzed at regular intervals during the night. Different species of animals behave differently when they dream. For example, dolphins dream with only one brain hemisphere at a time, possibly because they have one center to control their respiration, so they can swim even while they sleep. Cats sometimes twitch while they sleep, which has led to the theory that dreams might be useful for rehearsing complex sequences of movement, and may also explain why human infants dream so much.

● SLEEPLESS BRAINS

There are a number of interesting characteristics of paradoxical sleep that scientists still can't explain. Experiments have shown that if rats are prevented from sleeping, and in particular, from entering the paradoxical sleep phase, they will die in 2 to 3 weeks. The main cause of death appears to be that they become unable to regulate their body temperature. It has also been shown that if these deprived rats are suddenly allowed to enter paradoxical sleep right when they are about to die, they make a complete recovery, apparently without any permanent damage.

Humans deprived of sleep exhibit depression, hallucinations, and a diminished capacity for work. It is difficult to prevent humans, particularly those who are sleep deprived, from going into REM sleep. Although REM typically occurs

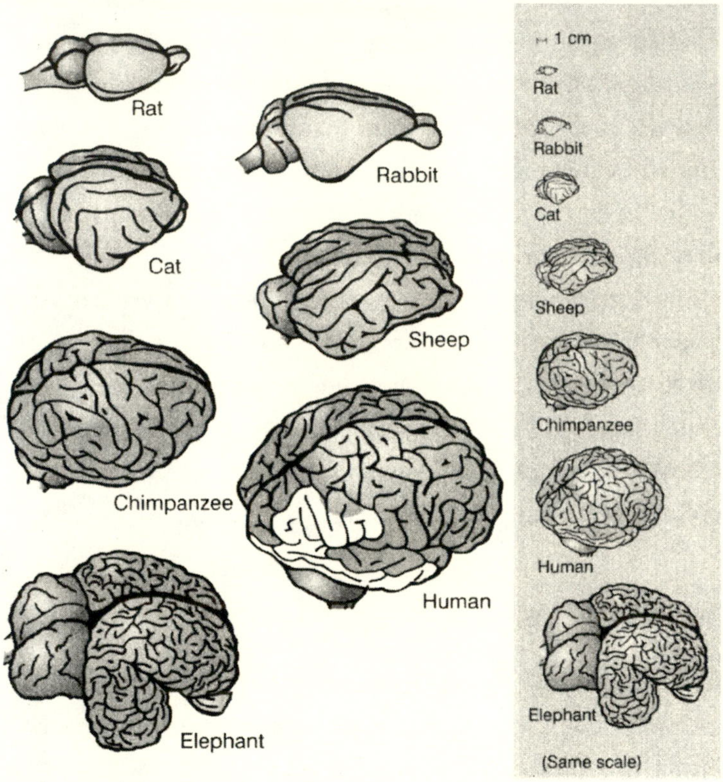

Figure 3.1 The brains of different mammals. The brain follows the same master plan in all mammals as shown above. The main differences between species are mostly in size (see right panel above) and folding patterns. The folds serve to extend the total amount of cortex, which can fit inside the narrow confines of the skull and, in particular, make it possible that the head can pass through the pelvic region at birth. The rat brain has very few folds, while rabbits and cats start to have more folds. The chimpanzee brain is remarkably similar to the human brain, which, contrary to what some might think, does not have the most complex folding patterns. Larger mammals such as elephants and whales have significantly more complex brain folding patterns than humans.

90 minutes after sleep begins, sleep-deprived humans go straight into REM, which lends more support to the idea that REM plays some important role in our lives. Although researchers do not know what this role is, some have proposed that sleep's main function is to consolidate memories, while others have suggested a link with the immune system. Experiments in which subjects are permitted to sleep for only a short time show that it is possible to temporarily skip sleep, although not without increased drowsiness during the day and, eventually, time spent making up the deficit. Given these consequences, it is probably worth questioning the wisdom of forcing people, such as doctors and truck drivers, into chronic sleep deprivation.

REASONABLE ABSURDITIES

When speaking of consciousness, we are usually more interested in its content than its states, such as waking and sleeping. This content includes life's pleasures and desires, of which social interactions—including our ability to empathize with others and appreciate their perspectives—play a significant role, as illustrated in the following joke: A kangaroo enters a bar and orders a single malt whiskey. The puzzled bartender serves the whiskey and says, "that will be $40." The kangaroo takes some money from his pouch and pays. From time to time, the bartender glances at the kangaroo slowly sipping his whiskey. Soon the bartender can no longer contain himself and says, "There are not many kangaroos around these parts." The kangaroo promptly replies, "It is hardly surprising when you are charging $40 for a whiskey." This joke, like many others, contains what could be called a *reasonable absurdity.* Although the joke contains many absurdities, such as the idea of English-speaking, whiskey-drinking kangaroos going to bars, only the kangaroo's answer to the bartender's question is a reasonable absurdity.

To get the joke, we have to combine knowledge of different things: bars, bartenders, kangaroos, single malt whiskey, and payment systems. As part of what could be loosely termed *social intelligence*, we have learned to assume that it is reasonable to buy single malt whiskey from a bartender in a bar. Our knowledge of natural history gives us typical kangaroo habitats and behaviors, which don't include, among other things, ordering a whiskey in a bar.

Different knowledge areas are important parts of the content of consciousness and may function in a modular fashion, similar to the parts of a Swiss Army knife. Some researchers, including the archaeologist Steven Mithen, have proposed that these two areas of knowledge—social intelligence and natural history—were separate in early hominids, and that humans are the first animals to be able to blend them. From an evolutionary perspective, this blending process has made us more successful than other animals. If our hominid ancestors were not sufficiently flexible to blend, they would not have been able to get the joke even if they had known about kangaroos, bars, and single malt whiskey.

Milk-Filled Breasts

Are metaphors such as modules and descriptions of Swiss Army knives adequate to explain the complex reality of the mind? Philosophers and cognitive psychologists such as Jerry Fodor and Steven Pinker have made much of the idea of the brain as a collection of many highly specialized modules. The idea of a modular brain is often used as an alternative to the earlier idea of the brain as a general, all-purpose learning machine. Evolutionary psychologists Leda Cosmides and John Tooby have adopted this idea of modules and searched for explanations of how these modules evolved. Much of their research concentrates on finding causes for how, under the demands and limitations of our environment, our brains have developed to the extent that they are able to understand language, discover cheaters in social situations, and even find lost infants and ease their access to milk-filled breasts.

Evolutionary explanations can be entertaining, but often the long, complex explanations that claim to trace our behavior to challenges of prehistoric climate and landscape are frighteningly similar to those in the British writer Rudyard Kipling's 1902 book, *Just So Stories*. These charming, well-known tales develop a more or less plausible story of how a certain attribute was created, such as how the leopard got its spots, the dromedary its hump, and the rhinoceros its wrinkled skin, as well as how the first letter was written and how the alphabet came into being. The problem with these types of evolutionary explanations is that it is not possible to carry out controlled experiments to test whether an explanation is really causal. For good reasons we are unable to repeat history to see what would have happened if the conditions had been different.

The modular brain metaphor does have some basis in reality, as the brain clearly consists of regions that carry out particular functions. For example, certain brain regions process sensory impressions that are brought together in other brain regions, and both types of regions can be described as modules because they are discrete units that interact to carry out a specific function. Although metaphors like modules and Swiss Army knives may work to help illuminate the brain's basic structure and some of its basic processes, the problem is that because we can describe most processes—brain or otherwise—as the interaction between modules, it is not clear that these metaphors provide us with anything special to help us understand the more complex functions of the brain. These metaphors also begin to break down when we try to describe how the discrete regions interact over time, how they generate higher mental constructs such as thoughts, and how they relate to the underlying neural structures.

THE BIOLOGY OF RELIGION

Religion follows the biological tracks of our evolutionary heritage and offers an understanding that is deeper and more sophisticated than the idea of "selfish genes" proposed by the English Darwinian fundamentalist Richard Dawkins. The purpose of our religious instinct is to maintain control over the uncontrollable and give meaning to enigmatic and perhaps even meaningless experiences. As such, the religious instinct as a meaning-making device is present across all human cultures, but takes many guises in addition to organized religion.

Although many people think of religion as a unique human trait that is closely linked to the deepest content of consciousness, there is now evidence for more of an evolutionary continuum. In the middle of the second century, the Greek orator Aelius Aristeides described how the God Asclepius told him in a dream that he would die within 3 days unless he made complex offerings, including sacrificing a sheep and "cutting off a part of his body to save the whole." During the same dream, Asclepius changed his mind and asked instead for Aristeides' ring, which of course, he was happy to offer rather than one of his precious body parts. Although Aristeides' dream may seem superstitious to many, even today people in numerous different cultures will ritualistically cut off a finger or part of finger when confronted with illness or the possibility of suffering.

Some animal species will also sacrifice a body part in order to preserve their lives. For example, animals that catch their legs in traps will chew them off to escape. This is not to say that foxes and humans use the same biological mechanisms. The desperate chewing off of a leg is very different from the conscious thoughts and actions underlying human ritual and narrative traditions. What we do share with other animals is an instinct for survival that's so strong that we will cut off a part to save the rest of our body, which is a reasonable response. But the action goes beyond reasonable when it's part of a ritual. As the link to the instrumental action, the link between cause and effect, gets lost over time, the action becomes exaggerated and demonstrative, and may eventually become ritualized, so that only the act in itself becomes important. This is how survival behavior can be promoted to ritual behavior.

It is difficult to see how human rituals and ideas would stem only from cultural learning, observations, empathy, or creativity. The facts that religious patterns are repeated across cultures, space, and time, and that we intuitively understand them, seem to reflect deeper evolutionary principles. Evolutionarily old brain structures, such as the periaqueductal gray, the amygdala, and the orbitofrontal cortex, are necessary to help control our emotional behavior, thus also our fight-or-flight behavior. Although few of us have been the victim of a predator, most of us can imagine how deeply terrifying it must be. Our aversion to uncontrollable panic has led us to construct a series of defense mechanisms to avoid it in our daily lives.

As always in nature, the sublime is not far from the absurd. One of the most violent reflexes against panic is involuntary defecation. In our daily lives, we have constructed a series of defense mechanisms to avoid uncontrollable panic, but in extreme situations such as a traffic accident or war, we become unable to control this reflex. Throughout history, this biological reflex has given rise to ritual. Thieves in Austria and Germany felt safe from detection and persecution if they left their excrement at the scene of the crime. In Greek religion, the symbol of panic in the dark, the goddess Hecate, is called *borborophorba*, "the eater of excrements."

The principle of offering "the part for whole" is perhaps even more telling when considering groups of humans. Perhaps the most well-known example is Jesus. This practice of saving everyone for the price of one life has become one of the central dogmas of Christianity, and can also be found as far back as the Babylonian creation myth, *Enuma elish*.

According to the Swiss classicist Walter Burkert, the question of religion cannot be reduced to either a self-governed expression of our genetic heritage, or a random culturally transmitted learning. He proposes that religion and sacrifice should be seen as a series of biological patterns of actions, reactions, and emotions linked to and detailed in ritual practice and verbal learning, with fear and punishment playing central roles.

BEHAVIOR WITHOUT PLEASURE AND DESIRE?

Russian American writer Isaac Asimov was a master at combining technological dreams with edgy prose that both anticipated and inspired the future. His stories are prophetic in their vision of a future in which robots assume boring and dangerous tasks so humans can concentrate on more important things. Unlike humans, whom Asimov portrays as irrational beings, most of his robots are governed solely by logic.

Asimov's stories raise an interesting question: Is it really possible to create complex human-like behavior without adding emotions, desires, and pleasures? Much evidence from the brain sciences suggests that to make conscious robots in our image, we would be well advised to imbue them with emotions. Although biological brains are more or less (often less) capable of solving logical problems, this should not be surprising as they have evolved primarily to survive and to reproduce, which does not always involve logic.

SUBJECTIVE PLEASURE

If we can hope to create a robot in our image, it seems that these robots would need similar systems for reward, pleasure, and desire in order to create consciousness content that truly corresponds to ours. Such artificially conscious beings are also likely to need bodies, because our consciousness is very much bounded by our physicality.

A very simple description of our understanding of the interplay between brain, body, and environment shows the brain integrating sensory impressions from the environment with physical states and needs, to allow for the best possible decisions and behavior. The integration includes the active processes of desire, pleasure, and emotion, which will take past experience and expectation into account to ultimately bring about at least two kinds of change: *External change* in the form of muscle movements, whether large-scale limb movements or speech (as already pointed out by the English neurophysiologist Charles Sherrington), and *Internal change* to our bodily organs, such as that seen in flight-or-fight behavior, which can cause changes in heart rhythm and in the production of sweat and gastric acids.

Both kinds of changes become part of the complex feedback systems that in turn cause changes in the functional organization of the brain in the form of learning, memories and thoughts, which help us continue to adapt our behavior in the future.

THE PRIVILEGE OF LANGUAGE

Information transfer between organisms is fundamental to all life. Throughout evolution, selection processes have allowed organisms to develop their special systems of communication, which are still limited by their sensory systems. We socially mirror ourselves in other people, and have an innate ability to represent and understand the behavior of others. We translate their behavior into our understanding of sensations, expectations, and goals, and use much of our time second-guessing their intentions, pleasures, desires, and motives. Although we don't know nearly enough about the details of this communication, other animals also can clearly communicate with each other and perhaps even sense the perspective of others.

Human language is one of the most advanced forms of communication we know of. It probably is also what we know the least about in terms of brain function, although scientists have recently discovered a link between the language areas of the human brain and the areas where mirror neurons have been found in monkey brains. Mirror neurons fire in the same way whether we execute an action ourselves or observe an action executed by another. From humans with brain damage, we know that certain areas of the brain, such as Broca's or Wernicke's, are more important for language than other brain areas. But we have yet to understand why language typically occurs on the brain's left side. We are also far from understanding how strongly epileptic children can have a whole hemisphere removed without much of a functional difference in their language skills.

Although we are likely to learn more about how the brain creates language, we will need brain scanners, such as magnetoencephalography (MEG), which can measure changes in the brain that occur over one thousandth of a second with a temporal resolution on the scale of milliseconds, to understand the complex mechanisms that underlie language. Our current ignorance is also the reason that we are far from creating robots that can carry on a meaningful conversation. In the meantime, it might be prudent to remember, as pointed out by Noam Chomsky, that we are likely to learn more about life and personality from novels than from scientific psychology.

● ● ● HAPPINESS LESSON

Don't stint on sleep or you may suffer. Though sleep is far from fully understood, it has been shown that regular sleep within somewhat flexible length parameters is necessary for our brains to function at their best. Without sleep we are much more prone to depression and anhedonia.

FURTHER READING

Our consciousness has recently become the object of disproportionate interest compared to altered conscious states and nonconscious processes in the human brain, which are just as important. Sleep is an example of an altered, yet mundane state of consciousness. One of the best books on this important topic is Lavie, P. (1996). *The Enchanted World of Sleep.* New Haven: Yale University Press.

Religion often involves trying to communicate with forces outside of our conscious control as eloquently described in Burkert, W. (1996). *The Creation of the Sacred. Tracks of Biology in Early Religions.* Cambridge, MA: Harvard University Press.

On a very deep level our consciousness is entangled with the efforts of giving meaning to that which may be random or meaningless. An excellent book that explores such problems within an evolutionary and cultural setting is Konner, M. (2002). *The Tangled Wing: Biological Constraints on the Human Spirit.* 2nd ed, New York, NY: Henry Holt.

4

EMOTIONS

Happiness, Fear, and Trembling

> Herein too may be felt the powerlessness of mere Logic . . . to resolve these problems which lie nearer to our hearts.
>
> George Boole (1815–1864)

> Le coeur a ses raisons que la raison ne connaît point.
>
> Blaise Pascal (1623–1662)

Roger is an overweight, red-cheeked man in his late thirties, with an easy laugh. Right now, however, he is not laughing. He has just lost a considerable amount of money in a game that most children would find easy.

The rules are simple. You have to choose between two geometric images on a computer screen. Choosing one of them will win you a large amount of money most of the time, whereas choosing the other will cost you. Once you have found the image that wins you the money, you have to keep choosing it until you consistently start to lose money. Then you have to switch to the other image to win money.

Roger knows he is losing money on the image he is choosing, but he cannot stop choosing it. He says he used to win money on this image, and even though he is aware that things have changed, he appears to be incapable of changing his behavior.

How is this possible? How can knowing the right course have little or no influence on Roger's subsequent decisions? A few years back, Roger suffered irreversible damage to the front part of his brain (the orbitofrontal cortex, located just over his eyeballs). Recent research suggests that this part of the human brain plays perhaps the most important role in decision making and emotional behavior. Invariably, damage to this part of the brain negatively affects behavior.

But it is not just patients with brain damage who make irrational decisions. Brain-imaging research seems to show that our decisions are rarely completely rational. In fact, many decisions are made on the basis of what are perhaps best described as emotional and nonconscious processes. A very interesting example of how nonconscious influences can drive decisions and behavior can be found in a social psychology experiment where male participants met the same young female interviewer either just before walking on or while on a swaying rope bridge. The men who met the interviewer on the bridge reported feeling a stronger physical attraction to her than those on a firmer footing. The changes in physical state were rationalized by the participants who claimed that the young woman, not the footbridge, was the most likely source.

Strong opinions shared by many people, such as those in politics, are most often based on deeply felt personal beliefs, and rarely on logic or rational arguments. Although these opinions can have damaging consequences, they can rarely be changed with more or better rational arguments, because the people's beliefs are the assumptions from which their rational analysis (if any) of the situation proceeds. Perhaps a better understanding of the underlying emotional processing in the human brain will help us deal more productively with the clash of such opinions and beliefs.

EMOTIONS AND SUBJECTIVE FEELINGS

Most people would probably agree that a life without emotions would be rather meaningless, as emotions are central to human life, and we closely associate them with the feeling of what it is to be conscious. If you think your emotions can be confusing and difficult to sort out and understand, you are correct. They have not been easy for even scientists to pin down. A brief look at the history of research in emotions gives an excellent indication of how scientists have struggled to quantify emotion.

Quantifying emotion is at least as difficult as quantifying the brain itself. Yet scientists have struggled for centuries to find appropriate metaphors to describe the functions of the brain. There is a long tradition of using the machine metaphor for the brain, and to update the metaphor with the newest, most advanced technology, water pumps, weaving looms, telephone centrals, and computers are among the machines that have been used.

Scientists have managed to divide the concept of emotion into two components: emotional states and feelings. Emotional states are physical, and so can be measured through physiological changes, such as involuntary responses including sweating and elevated heart rate. Feelings are more psychological, defined as the subjective experience of emotion. In other words, feelings are what it is *like* subjectively to experience an emotional state. Although there is not a lot of research on the more subject experience of feelings, scientists have made great advances in determining which brain areas are involved in producing and representing emotional states.

Western philosophers and scientists have traditionally tried to use purely rational means to investigate our thought processes, and so cognition and emotion have been regarded as separate areas. For the greater part of the twentieth century, most scientific research focused on cognition, but ignored emotion. Nonetheless, some important advances were made by pioneering individuals, such as Charles Darwin, who examined the evolution of emotional responses and facial expressions. Darwin's work led to the important insight into evolution that emotions enable an organism to make adaptive responses to salient stimuli in the environment, thus enhancing its chances of survival, and that emotions and the associated subjective experience must have therefore been selected by evolution.

Bodily Emotions

It seems natural to view emotions as internal reactions to external stimuli, but in the 1880s, we moved away from this view when the American psychologist William James and the Danish physiologist Carl Lange independently proposed the idea that emotional experience is the perception of physiological changes, not a response to a stimulus. The James–Lange theory suggests that we do not run from the bear because we are afraid, but that we *become* afraid because we run. The theory does not explain why we start to run in the first place, but only that we become afraid when we run. It also favors the body over the brain.

Some scientists have remained skeptical of these so-called bodily theories of emotion. William Cannon, for example, wrote a detailed critique of the James–Lange theory in the 1920s and showed that surgical disruption of the peripheral nervous system in dogs did not eliminate emotional responses as the James–Lange theory predicted. Further investigations suggested that bodily states must be accompanied by cognitive appraisal for an emotion to occur. When running from the bear, one has to actively appraise why the body has been put in a state of alert before being able to experience the conscious feeling of fear. Scientists have, however, still not fully resolved the basic question of the extent to which bodily states influence emotion and feelings. The James–Lange theory was resurrected in the 1970s by the American neuroanatomist Walla Nauta, and then again in the 1990s—to far more popular acclaim—by the American-Portuguese neurologist Antonio Damasio. According to these theories, the body helps shape the *decision* about what to do about the bear running after us, rather than the *experience* of running scared.

Among the objections to the bodily theories of emotion is that they do not specify what constitutes emotional stimuli.

Why is it that bears and not, say, tables give rise to strong emotions? Signals from the body are also inherently noisy, so it is not clear whether people can distinguish the different emotions. Are the butterflies in our stomach a sign of joy, worry, or just something we ate? Another potential problem is that animals and humans with severe spinal cord damage appear to have normal emotions. As the bodily theories claim that the signals indicating emotions travel through the spinal cord, this finding is a real problem for them. However, it has also been argued that emotions are constituted largely of visceral and endocrine responses, rather than through the spinal cord. The orbitofrontal cortex certainly has the ability to receive and integrate visceral sensory signals and then influence ongoing behavior. Although it is not clear how this information is integrated, it remains possible that these signals play a significant role in decision making and emotion.

Although there is a lot of uncertainty about the general relationship between the body and emotion, the successful use of various beta-blockers in alleviating stage fright, anxiety, and panic attacks in musicians and other world-class performers has made it clear that the body plays some role in how emotions are regulated. As a result, some have suggested that the role of the body in emotion is perhaps more akin to an amplifier than a generator.

Investigating Emotional States

The development of experimental paradigms for the reliable testing of emotion in animals and humans has also taken many detours. In their investigations of emotion, neuroscientists have concentrated on understanding the brain structures that control rewards and punishments. The basic learning process is called *conditioning*, and much psychological research has been dedicated to understanding its underlying principles.

Although the Russian neurophysiologist Ivan Petrovich Pavlov did not start the research on conditioning, he carried out the most systematic research on salivation in hungry dogs, for which he received the Nobel Prize in 1904. Pavlov's dogs learned that food always followed the tick of a metronome, so they started to salivate at the sound. Pavlov's ground-breaking research is the basis for what has become known as classical conditioning. Classical conditioning is a very simple form of learning, but there are many more complicated learning processes. An important class of learning process was discovered by the American psychologist Edward Thorndike in 1895. Thorndike's animals had to take a certain action, such as pressing a lever, to obtain food or leave their cage. He found that although it takes a long time for the animals to find the correct behavior, once they learn it, the behavior becomes automated. These learning processes were further investigated and classified by another American psychologist, Burrhus Frederic Skinner, the father of behaviorism. He classified the process of *instrumental or operant conditioning*, in which food only becomes visible after the animal carries out the correct behavior. This is different from classical Pavlovian conditioning in which the food is always visible during the learning.

Behaviorism was for many years the mainstay of experimental psychology, and during this time, the brain got no respect. For Skinner, the brain was as an uninteresting black box. His only interest was in the behavior of animals, where responses slavishly follow stimuli, and where all behavior was completely flexible, given the right reward schedule. Much subsequent research has shown that the original tenets of behaviorism were oversimplified, if not plain wrong. The species-specific features of the brain matter very much and make all the difference for its learning potential. Subjective experience does not depend in any simple way on stimuli and responses, and even the most cunning reward schedules cannot change some species-specific behaviors (Figure 4.1).

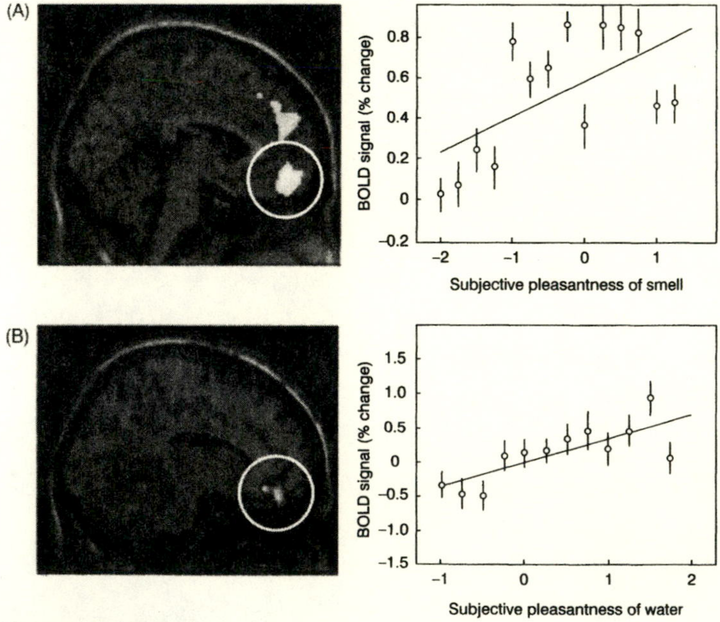

Figure 4.1 (Contd)

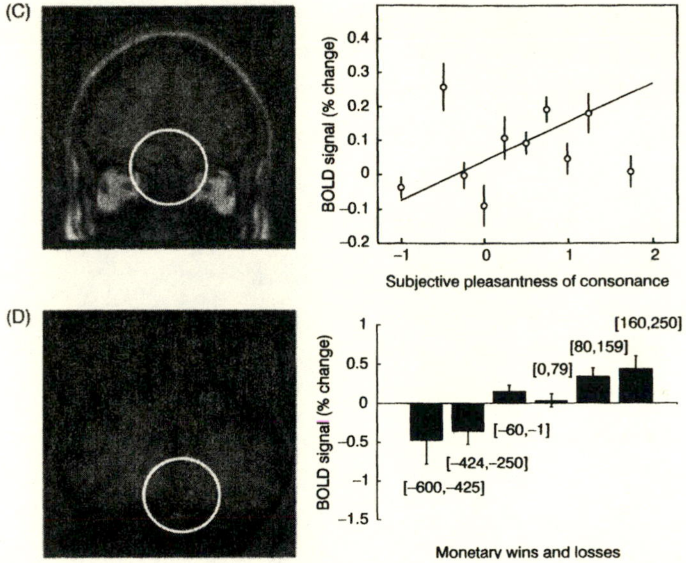

Figure 4.1 Valence coding in medial orbitofrontal cortex (OFC). (A) The activity in medial OFC correlates with the subjective ratings of pleasantness in an experiment with three pleasant and three unpleasant odors. (B) Similarly, the activity in medial OFC was also correlated with the subjective pleasantness ratings of water in a thirst experiment. A correlation in a very similar part of medial OFC was found with the pleasantness of other pure tastants used in the experiment (not shown). (C) This corresponded to the findings in an experiment investigating taste and smell convergence and consonance, which found that activity in the medial OFC was correlated to subjective consonance ratings. (D) Even higher-order rewards such as monetary reward was found to correlate with activity in the medial OFC.

THE FEAR CENTER?

Conditioning experiments are nonetheless important for offering insights into some of the fundamental forms of learning. Neuroscientists have learned a great deal by studying brain activity with experimental paradigms adapted from behaviorism. In one type of experiment, an animal must learn that only certain stimuli will lead to a reward, while other stimuli will bring about punishment. This learning is sufficiently important for the survival of the animal as it leads to those mental and physical states called emotions. One of the most successful paradigms in emotion research has been fear conditioning, in which an auditory conditioned stimulus is paired with a shock to the foot or paw, as the case may be. As the animal hears a tone and receives a shock, it eventually learns the association. By removing parts of the rat brain in conjunction with this experiment, scientists have worked out which brain structures are important for fear. The fear-conditioning paradigm has been very successful in creating a scientific model of emotion and in firmly establishing the field of emotion research.

Much of this research has indicated that a structure called the *amygdala* plays a central role in the rat brain fear system. In fact, removal of all or select parts of the amygdala can abolish the fear reaction in rats. The amygdala is not actually a homogeneous brain structure, but rather a collection of at least 14 anatomically distinct nuclei. So much neuroscientific research has focused on elucidating the full role of the amygdala in fear that it has become known as *the fear center.* However, some research has indicated that the amygdala can be activated by both positive and negative stimuli, so it is unlikely that the amygdala is concerned only with fear. It has also become clear that the amygdala might be very important for rodents, but as a lot has happened to the structure of the brain on the evolutionary path to higher primates, it is unclear how important the amygdala is for us.

Some scientists have proposed that the amygdala obtains information about significant stimuli in the environment earlier than other brain areas in the cortex. This allows the brain to send early warning signals via the amygdala to the rest of the brain and the body. If we were to suddenly notice something that at first glance looked like a snake, our brain and body would be able to react quickly, but essentially nonconsciously. We are able to have the emotional fear reactions immediately via the amygdala, and so we become aware that we are fearful before we are aware of what made us fearful. Reacting quickly to dangerous stimuli has probably provided an evolutionary advantage, so these essentially nonconscious reactions could possibly explain why James and Lange proposed that the body controls emotions. This scenario does not work in the snake example, however, because the information is first processed in the brain, and then the amygdala alerts the body. It is clear that this confusion over the path that emotion takes is yet another good illustration of how little insight we have into our own brain processing.

WANTING AND LIKING

In parallel studies during the 1950s, Canadian psychologists James Olds and Peter Milner found that rats would repeatedly press levers to receive tiny jolts of current through electrodes implanted deep within their brains. When this brain stimulation was targeted at certain areas of the brain, the rats would repeatedly press the lever—even up to 2000 times per hour. In fact, they would stop almost all other normal behaviors, including feeding, drinking, and having sex. The findings seemed to suggest that Olds and Milner had discovered the pleasure center in the brain. One of the main chemicals aiding neural signaling in these regions is dopamine, and so it was quickly dubbed the brain's "pleasure chemical." Human studies during the 1960s by the American psychiatrist Robert Heath tried to take advantage of these findings in some ethically questionable experiments on mentally ill patients. They even implanted electrodes to try to cure homosexuality. Although the researchers also found compulsive lever pressing in some patients, it is not clear from these patients' subjective reports that the electrodes did indeed cause real pleasure.

Recent work by Kent Berridge indicates that the electrodes may have activated the anatomical regions that are involved in desire rather than pleasure. When Berridge manipulated rodents' dopamine levels, he found that although they did try to get to the reward much more quickly than normal rodents, their facial expressions remained unchanged. From his earlier work, Berridge knew that this is not what would be expected if dopamine really elicits pleasure. In another set of elegant experiments, Berridge found that stimulation of specific parts of the rat brain contribute to the hedonic impact of sweetness, food, and drug rewards. He was able to show that there are hedonic maps in the nucleus accumbens, which receives much of its information from the orbitofrontal cortex.

How can we explain these findings? In Chapter 5, we will see how the brain carries out the early sensory processing. Suffice to say here that an integral part of all sensory stimuli is our hedonic experience of its pleasant and unpleasant aspects. Of course, these hedonic experiences come only later in brain processing, but they do ultimately help us decide on the best possible actions for navigating complex physical and social environments. Early theories of motivation proposed that this hedonic behavior is controlled by need states, which unfortunately does not explain why people continue to eat food when they are full. This behavior was addressed by incentive-motivation theories that found that hedonic behavior is mostly determined by the incentive value of a stimulus or its capacity to function as a reward. According to these theories, need states, such as hunger, are still important, but work only indirectly on the incentive value of the stimulus. This is why sweet foods taste less pleasant when you are full compared with when you are hungry, and you can be full enough to leave your main course, but still have room for dessert.

Berridge therefore proposed a distinction between the dual aspects of reward: hedonic impact and incentive salience. Hedonic impact is the *liking* or pleasure related to the reward. Incentive salience is the *wanting* or desire for the reward. Experiments by Berridge and others suggest that there is a dissociation in terms of both the brain regions and the neurochemical substances that mediate pleasure and desire. The dopamine system appears to encode desire, while the opioid system—which contains the brain's own natural morphine-like compounds—is closer to pleasure (Figure 4.2).

EMOTION AND FEELINGS IN HUMANS

Until the advent of neuroimaging, research on human brains was limited to patients with lesion sites. Scientists have investigated emotions in animals, but it is not clear

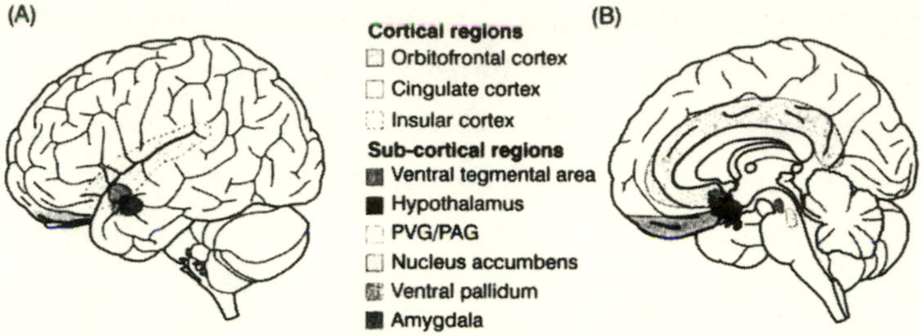

Figure 4.2 Pleasure regions. The figure shows the human brain seen from the side (A) and split in the middle (B) overlaid with the approximate location of the important brain structures of the pleasure brain. These include cortical areas such as the orbitofrontal (light gray), the cingulate (stippled) and the insular cortices (buried between the prefrontal and temporal lobes, hatched) as well as subcortical areas such as the ventral tegmental area in the brainstem (medium gray), hypothalamus (dark gray), periventricular gray/periaqueductal gray (PVG/PAG, dotted), nucleus accumbens (medium hatched), ventral pallidum (stippled) and the amygdala (dark gray).

whether and how this research transfers to humans, especially given the subjective nature of conscious feelings, which have not been proven to exist in other animals. However, early cross-cultural behavioral studies showed that there might be an innate, biological basis for emotional experience. The American psychologist Paul Ekman demonstrated that facial expressions of emotion are universally recognized across cultures. Analyses of emotion terms in the world's major languages have enabled researchers to develop a list of fundamental emotions that may be the basic building blocks for our entire emotional repertoire. Seven emotions have been proposed: anger, disgust, fear, sadness, joy, shame, and guilt. We still don't know whether each of these emotions is really distinct, or whether they all line up on a continuum, as they all appear to be produced by shared brain mechanisms.

Research into the nature of emotion has been slow, with negative emotions, such as fear and disgust, engendering more inquiry than investigation of positive emotions such as joy. Work on positive emotions has been hampered by the fact that they are much more difficult to induce experimentally than negative emotions.

The case of Phineas Gage was one of the first to link the brain's frontal regions with human emotion. Gage was a railway engineer whose frontal lobes, including his orbitofrontal cortex, were penetrated when an explosion caused a metal rod to be shot through his head. Although Gage survived, according to the scant evidence available, his personality and emotional processing were changed completely. Roger (from the beginning of this chapter) and other patients with damage to the front parts of the brain, in particular the orbitofrontal cortex, have exhibited important changes in their emotion, personality, behavior, and social conduct. Such patients often show lack of affect and responsibility, as well as generally inappropriate social behavior.

Results from neuroimaging and lesion studies in humans and other higher primates have indicated that several interconnected brain structures work together to process and mediate emotion. An early but pervasive idea was that the *limbic* system mediated emotions. Subsequent research shows such ideas to be oversimplified, and points instead to the amygdala and the cingulate cortex. The most recent evidence has confirmed that the most likely candidates among human brain structures for the processing and mediation of emotion and feelings are the orbitofrontal cortex, the cingulate cortex, and the amygdala. A significant role is played by the orbitofrontal cortex, a brain region that connects to both the opioid and dopamine systems and contains regions that correlate with subjective reports of pleasure. Neuroimaging of normal subjects has also shown that all of the primary sensory information is processed in the orbitofrontal cortex.

CHRONIC-PAIN RELIEF

Using electrodes to directly stimulate the brain has made a remarkable comeback. The case of Robert is an excellent example of the power of this technique. Robert's leg was amputated, following a fall. His aura of calm belies the suffering that drove him into a deep depression and almost to suicide. After the amputation, Robert's doctors tried to alleviate the excruciating pain in his phantom leg with many different kinds of pain treatments, but nothing worked. Finally, as Robert contemplated how best to end it all, he heard of the Oxford neurosurgeon Tipu Aziz.

Aziz and his team have pioneered the use of deep brain stimulation for chronic pain and movement disorders, such as Parkinson's disease. Precise anatomical information from brain imaging allows Aziz to precisely implant electrodes into any part of the brain. Animal experiments have shown that chronic pain can be reduced by stimulation of the thalamus and a region in the upper brainstem called the *periaqueductal gray.* Aziz performs the surgery while the patient is awake, so that when the electrodes are in place, the neurosurgeons can activate them and obtain direct reports from the patient on the effects of the stimulation (Figure 4.3).

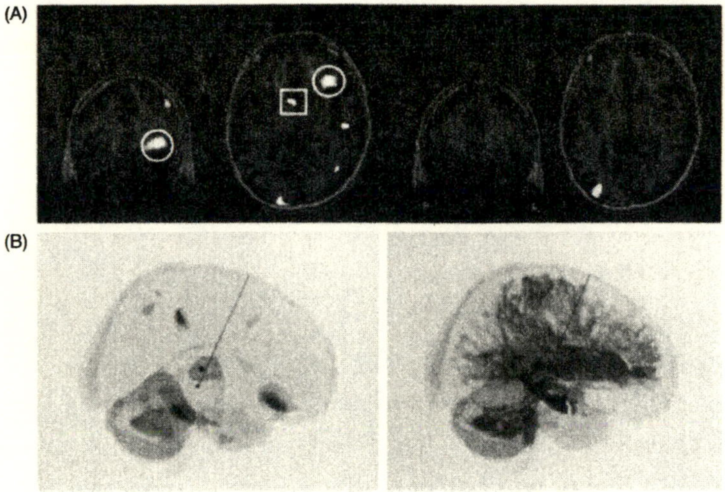

Figure 4.3 Deep brain stimulation (DBS). We used magnetoencephalography (MEG) to measure the effects of deep brain stimulation in the brainstem for the treatment of Robert's phantom limb pain. (A) When subjective pain relief was obtained, there were significant activity increases in the left mid-anterior orbitofrontal cortex (left). Activity in these brain regions was not found when DBS was turned off, resulting in significantly more pain (right). (B) The resulting pleasure is also shown in a three-dimensional rendering of the human brain with the implanted electrode (left). The significant increases in activity are shown in shades of gray, while other landmark brain structures can be seen including the thalamus, cerebellum, and brainstem. This result fits with the anatomical connectivity from the electrode as shown in the figure at the right, with the probabilistic tractography presented in different colors from more (lighter gray) to less significant (darker gray).

Robert was thus fully awake when Aziz and his team implanted the four electrodes in his upper brainstem. At first, the stimulation did not seem to ease the pain; in fact, it became worse. But then, as if by magic, Robert said he felt a sudden calm descend. Where did that pain go? The pain was still there somewhere, but it was suddenly much more bearable. The surgical team had just changed the frequency and electrode of the stimulation, which seemed to make all the difference. When the stimulator was turned off, Robert reported that the pain came back almost immediately. Some days later, a long-lasting battery was implanted over Robert's right breast muscle and connected permanently to the deep brain electrodes. Through a remote control, the doctors can change the frequency, pulse width, and power of the stimulation to obtain the best possible results. Robert is now back to doing the things he enjoys and has even started working again. The effects of deep brain stimulation are even more striking when applied to patients with Parkinson's disease. In fact, some of these symptoms can be switched on and off in a way that looks almost magical to the untrained eye.

Deep brain stimulation is obviously not magical, but the result of careful scientific experimentation. Although scientists are getting amazing results, they still don't understand how different brain regions contribute to pain or its relief. They are particularly puzzled by how stimulation of certain deep brain regions drives activity in wider brain regions, such as the neocortex and subcortical regions. My research team recently shed some light on this matter. We scanned Robert using a technique called *magnetoencephalography* that allowed us to map how his brain activity had changed as a result of deep brain stimulation. We found significant changes in Robert's brain activity in a network that contains the regions of brain associated with emotion, including the mid-anterior orbitofrontal and subgenual cingulate cortices.

Given the complexity of the human brain, it is unlikely that we will find a single center for pain relief or even pleasure, but one day we may be able to help patients with chronic pain, and even with depression, not necessarily with deep brain stimulation, but through the information gained through basic research on patients like Robert.

The neuroscience of happiness and well-being is still in its infancy. As shown in this book, much of the focus of research has thus far been on two related but perhaps somewhat distant cousins: desire and pleasure. Some of this research has focused on understanding how and why desire and pleasure turn malignant. Many of these processes are shaped in early childhood. A good example is provided by the Danish poet Henrik Nordbrandt in his memoirs of a horrible childhood in Denmark in the 1950s, in which a rare consolation was the occasional loving care from his grandparents. In one of the most horrific passages, Nordbrandt recounts how his mother, inspired by a book on child rearing by a renowned psychologist, and in keeping with the times, avoided touching him any more than absolutely necessary. One day she went for a walk with young Henrik in the pram, sat down to relax on a bench, and as usual, left Henrik in the pram. She started chatting with a nearby pair of old ladies who told her that even if it was against the fashion of the day, they were convinced that the child would come to no harm if he were picked up. The young mother considered this, but chose to stick to what she saw as scientifically proven advice.

Even the experts had come to doubt the advice, because at that time, scientists in Wisconsin were at work on a series of experiments that would change psychologists' view on child development and in particular, the importance of early affection. But these insights had a very high price for all of the scientists involved. We will look into these controversial experiments before delving deeper into the depths of despair and madness of the human mind.

HARMFUL MATERNAL LOVE

The research program in Wisconsin was led by the American psychologist Harry Harlow, who eventually became synonymous with this research. Harlow was a very capable and energetic scientist with a complex personality. Unfortunately he was also a workaholic who ended up deeply alcoholic, with several severe depressions and subsequent confinement in psychiatric wards.

Harlow spent 40 years in a position at the University of Wisconsin, where he carried out the research with rhesus monkeys that changed the scientific view of love and, in particular, maternal love. Behaviorism, the prevailing fashion of those days, claimed to be able to explain all human behavior from rat models. But unlike most universities at the time, the University of Wisconsin did not use rats, so Harlow was challenged early on by behaviorists to show whether there was any behavior that could not be described by similar behavior in rats. It is characteristic for Harlow in his early career that he lacked the necessary self-confidence to tackle this directly. But it is also characteristic that Harlow did come up with the good answer that rat models of reading might be a bit of a challenge.

Surrogate Mothers

Harlow's research can be seen as an important confrontation with behaviorism in three main phases. The first phase was aimed at the prevailing view of behaviorism that all learning in animals is only governed by reward. Harlow's research showed that curiosity also drove monkeys, which became motivated by tasks simply because the tasks were interesting. The monkeys became quickly adept at what is best characterized as strategic thinking.

The second phase started by accident. The imported monkeys were prone to serious illness, which made the research difficult, so Harlow and his team decided to start a breeding program for monkeys and, to minimize the risk of infection, to isolate newborn babies immediately after birth. Harlow immediately noticed that the isolated babies developed very differently from normal monkeys and became deeply asocial.

This was the beginning of a large research program that tried to investigate why a newborn monkey became attached to the mother. At the time, the standard answer from behaviorism was that the mother gave the newborn reward in the form of food. So scientists decided that it was more important to keep the newborns sterile and infection free than to give them the physical contact, which was seen as unnecessary and perhaps even detrimental to their mental health. The argument went that too much physical contact would render them incompetent and inert as adults, and it was undoubtedly such arguments that the mother of Henrik Nordbrandt had read.

For a surrogate mother, the researchers gave the isolated baby monkeys a rag doll. The monkeys became very attached to the dolls; experiments showed that even when the monkeys had to choose between the rag doll and a similar-looking metal doll that rewarded them with food, the monkeys chose the rag doll and minimized their time with the metal doll. In other words, it appeared that the development of emotional links had little to do with a reward measured in calories, strong evidence against the simple reward philosophy of behaviorism. But even when using the rag doll as their companion, the monkeys still became deeply asocial. This sparked the third, very dark phase of Harlow's research. What is it that creates asocial behavior? Is it the isolation from the mother or from other monkeys? Can early emotional damage be repaired? The researchers tried to answer these questions by performing rather cruel experiments. In one experiment, a spray of cold water from the rag doll punished the monkey for clinging to its surrogate mother. This caused the monkey to cling even harder to the rag doll, which is not unlike the behavior seen in some domestic abuse.

This kind of animal research is very difficult to defend ethically. Even worse treatment came in later experiments (when Harlow was severely hit by depression and alcoholism at the time when his second wife was dying from cancer). The researchers tried to demonstrate how isolated and asocial female monkeys make poor mothers, but these monkeys had trouble reproducing normally. To solve this, the researchers invented a "rape rack" (as it was called by Harlow), which kept the female monkey tied down, while the males would rape her. Not surprisingly, the raped asocial female monkeys made highly incompetent mothers. One must question why it was necessary for the female monkeys to suffer.

In the same way, it seems inexcusable that the researchers attempted to induce depression in monkeys by isolating them for months in what Harlow called the "pit of despair." Monkeys who were otherwise normal became deeply antisocial after spending time in the pit. Later research showed that these monkeys could be helped back from the brink of depression by gentle contact with very young monkeys.

From this account, it will appear that Harlow came to play a demonic lead role in what resembles a horror movie about a scientist for whom the ends come to justify the means. (As a consequence of the reaction to the kinds of experiments carried out by Harlow and other contemporary researchers, animal experimentation is now more strictly controlled to minimize the suffering of the animals.) But while the conclusions obtained from Harlow's animal research can seem patently obvious today, this was not the case when the research was carried out.

More recent research on the emotional brain has shown that humans and other animals need social and emotional nurturing. This is amplified by close physical contact that helps reward systems to develop. One of our most important tasks of the twenty-first century must be to make sure that Harlow's hard-earned knowledge is not forgotten and to help improve the experience of childhood.

EMOTIONAL DAMAGE

The emotional and social problems following brain damage can be rather subtle, so although they may remain undiagnosed, they can cause serious problems for relatives and friends who have to live with what may still be radical changes in the personality of someone close to them. Fundamental to human social and emotional learning is our remarkably flexible behavior. Brain-damaged patients, like Roger at the beginning of this chapter, have lost the flexibility to understand when their options reverse. Normal patients, however, were able to track the reward value of the stimuli, and so understand when their options reversed. We found that the orbitofrontal cortex was clearly involved, but there was an interesting dissociation between the parts of the orbitofrontal cortex that were used. Brain activity in the medial orbitofrontal cortex was correlated with the monetary gains, while activity in the lateral orbitofrontal cortex was correlated with the losses. This distinction demonstrates that our brain keeps close track of losses and wins of even abstract rewards such as money. As we saw earlier, these results are closely related to the kind of social reversal learning that is central for shaping social interactions.

Although conscious appraisal of emotion is important for emotional expression, many emotional stimuli appear to be processed at a nonconscious level, only to become available later at a conscious level. Nonetheless, it is clear that emotions are evolutionarily important for animals in preparing for appropriate actions. The evolution of conscious feelings could be adaptive, because they allow us to consciously appraise our emotions and actions, and subsequently to learn to manipulate them appropriately. Emotion may be one of evolution's most productive breakthroughs, constantly reminding us that we are still animals at heart, but endowed with the possibility of conscious appraisal and enhanced control of our lives. A better understanding of emotions will help us function better with other people, which is perhaps the most emotionally intelligent road to happiness (Figure 4.4).

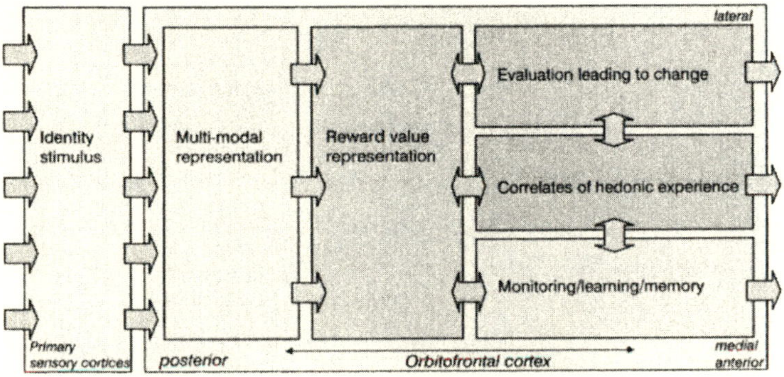

Figure 4.4 Pleasure model. Making sense of sensation involves hedonic evaluative processes that can help guide our behavior. The figure shows how this is thought to take place in the orbitofrontal cortex. On the left, sensory information arrives from the periphery to the primary sensory cortices, where the stimulus identity is decoded into stable cortical representations. This information is then conveyed for further multimodal integration in the posterior parts of the orbitofrontal cortex. The reward value of the reinforcer is assigned in more anterior parts of the orbitofrontal cortex from where it can then be used to influence subsequent behavior (in lateral parts of the anterior orbitofrontal cortex with connections to anterior cingulate cortex), stored for valence/learning/memory (in medial parts of the anterior orbitofrontal cortex), and made available for subjective hedonic experience (in mid-anterior orbitofrontal cortex). The reward value and the subjective hedonic experience can be modulated by hunger and other internal states. In addition, there is important reciprocal information flowing between the various regions of the orbitofrontal cortex and other brain regions.

● ● ● HAPPINESS LESSONS

Never insist on complete rationality, from yourself or others, because emotion is built into our decision making.

Desire and pleasure are not the same. If the things and activities you pursue do not, on reflection, bring you pleasure, it's time to reconsider your desires.

Physical contact and emotional affection are crucial in the emotional development of infants and children.

Liking and wanting in the brain

Scientific studies of pleasure has shown that liking, wanting, and learning are linked in the brain. Pleasure can be measured in other animals as reactions of "liking," "wanting," and "learning," where the quotation marks indicate that these are behavioral reactions in animals rather than everyday conscious human experiences.

Stimulating specific subregions of the brains of animals and humans can directly change the pleasure and desire. Research has also shown how some neurotransmitters play important roles for liking and wanting. Dopamine is more closely linked with "wanting" than with "liking," which instead appears to depend on the opiate system.

Pleasure does not necessarily follow the fulfillment of desire. If desire and wanting take over completely, the pleasure may well disappear. Animals and humans can become dependent not only on self-stimulation of the brain but also on drugs. While this may initially give them some pleasure, this often disappear with time. The learning processes involved can create strong addictions which can be very difficult to get rid of.

FURTHER READING

Emotion and feelings are exciting topics to research, which has developed quite a bit since Darwin's very readable book from 1872: Darwin (1872). *The Expression of the Emotions in Man and Animals.* Chicago: University of Chicago Press.

Emotion research in other animals is well described in these three books:

LeDoux, J.E. (1996). *The Emotional Brain.* New York, NY: Simon and Schuster.

Panksepp, J. (1999). *Affective Neuroscience.* Oxford: Oxford University Press.

Ekman, P. & Davidson, R. J. (1994). *The Nature of Emotion: Fundamental Questions.* New York, NY: Oxford University Press.

The science of pleasures and desires is remarkably sparse, but we are trying to remedy the situation in our forthcoming book: Kringelbach, M.L. & Berridge, K.C. (2008). *Pleasures of the Brain.* New York, NY: Oxford University Press.

5

SENSATION

Making Sense

> Food is an important part of a balanced diet.
>
> Fran Lebowitz (1950–)

> Si tu pouvais savoir tout ce que je vois! tout ce que je sens! tout ce que j'entends dans tes cheveux! Mon âme voyage sur le parfum comme l'âme des autres hommes sur la musique.
>
> Charles Baudelaire (1821–1867)

Our brains are firmly anchored in sensory inputs, so it should not be surprising that the worst kind of torture does not aim to inflict as much pain as possible, but to rob the victim of the ability to sense the surrounding world. Under such torture, most people very quickly lose their sanity, because without constant sensory inputs, the brain stops making sense. Our senses form the basis of our subjective experience, and we obtain the most fundamental pleasure through seeing, hearing, smelling, tasting, and touching the world around us. The brain is constantly trying to integrate the sensations it receives from the eyes, ears, nose, mouth, and skin, and then predict what will happen next, which is its most important job after making sense of the world. The senses influence how the brain represents the environment, and this representation is the basis for how we act in the world. The relative evolutionary success of humans may be partly due to our ability to use our sensory impressions to make predictions about the world and correct our own and others' behavior accordingly. If we pay attention to our senses, they offer us the possibility for more intelligent action. Before we venture further on our journey into the pleasures of the association cortices, however, we will need a firmer grasp of how these sensory inputs are initially processed.

SENSORY INPUTS

We are all familiar with the pleasant expectations generated by a table full of good food, or the immediate disappointment when a bitten potato chip does not give forth the expected crispy sound. The more basic our needs are, the more they involve a larger number of our sensory components. Our most basic and important needs—food and sex—heavily involve all of them. Sensory inputs come to the brain from our primary sensory organs (eyes, ears, nose, mouth, and skin), where there are receptors with many different properties. They convert sensory input to neural activity.

It is not entirely accurate to state that we only have five senses. The five senses that were classified by Aristotle can be further subdivided into other senses depending on which sensory receptors are being used. For example, taste receptors on the tongue react to the chemical compounds of sweet, sour, bitter salt, and umami; touch receptors react to pressure, pain, and temperature. But the classical view of five senses is important because those are the senses we are most aware of.

In terms of evolutionary history, taste, smell, and touch were probably the first senses to develop, while both sight and hearing are more recent. Sight and hearing work over longer distances, whereas taste, smell, and touch work best at short distances. Taste and smell are both chemical senses that give us information about the food that gives us the energy to live. Even primitive organisms have corresponding chemical senses that help them discover potential problems with food before it is consumed.

Our brains work in such a way that sensory information first shows up in brain areas where it is largely independent of an internal state, such as hunger. The information is then relayed to secondary areas where it is integrated with sensory information coming from the body, and may lead to a change in behavior (Figure 5.1). The first representation of sensory input has to remain independent of our general state to allow the most flexible behavior. If this were not the case, in the extreme it could mean that we would be unable to distinguish between various taste inputs when we are no longer hungry. Information about hunger and satiation is instead made available only in the secondary cortical areas, which allows satiation to be selective for only certain taste inputs,

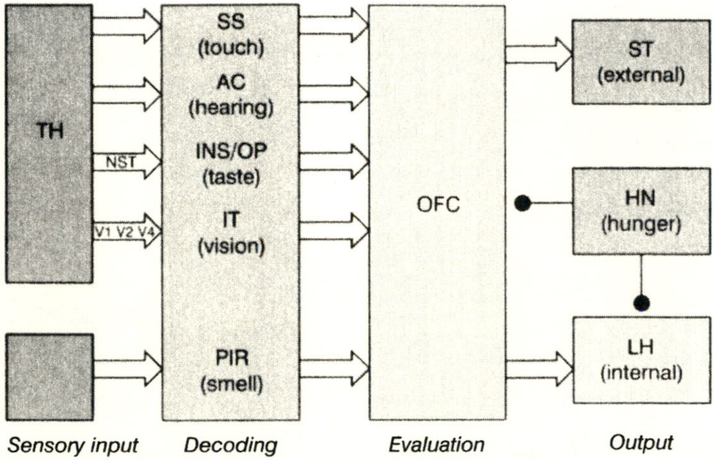

Figure 5.1 Decoding of sensation. The figure shows a model of how and where the brain decodes sensory input from the five senses. The sensory receptors for the five senses send electrical impulses to the primary sensory regions of the brain via the thalamus (TH)—except for smell. Touch is decoded in the somatosensory cortex (SS), hearing in the auditory cortex (AC), taste in nucleus solitaris (NST) in the brainstem and in insular/opercular cortex (INS/OP), while vision is decoded in the primary and higher visual areas (V1, V2, V4, IT). Smell is decoded in the primary olfactory regions in the piriform cortex (PIR) at the junction between temporal and frontal regions. The processed sensory inputs are then sent to other brain regions, in particular for integration and evaluation in the orbitofrontal cortex (OFC), where they can be modulated by internal states such as hunger via the hypothalamus (HN). The evaluated signals can then come to influence internal states through the lateral hypothalamus (LH) and external motor behavior through the striatum (ST).

which in turn facilitates adaptive behavior. From an evolutionary point of view, selective satiation lets us obtain a sufficiently varied diet. It has been proposed that this principle also holds true for sex.

Another important property of sensory inputs is that if they don't occur within certain physiological limits, we don't notice them until they become painful. For example, very cold or warm sensory inputs are often perceived as painful, depending on our core body temperature. Pain thus exists, at least in part, as a control mechanism to prevent damage to the organism.

Taste

Consuming food is the most important activity for animals to sustain life, and is, as a result, closely tied to our emotions and is one of the most important factors of our sense of well-being. With the abundance of food in the West, most of us do not have to think much about where our next meal is coming from, which makes it easy to forget how important food has been in the development of human cultures. The challenges of maintaining stable food sources in a variety of climates have been a driving force in the development of higher brain functions for all mammals. The relative sophistication of foraging in higher primates compared to other mammals indicates that significant parts of our large brains are dedicated to the required motivational, emotional, and cognitive processing, and that the mental processes related to food intake may underlie other higher functions.

When most people speak of the taste of food, they mean a combination of its taste, smell, and structure. Of these three qualities, smell is almost always the most dominant. Having a cold or holding your nose while eating will significantly reduce the sensory pleasure of food. However, from the brain's perspective, there are clear differences in the three sensory qualities, with taste receptors found primarily on the tongue, smell receptors in the nose, and structure receptors in the mouth, but not on the tongue (Figure 5.2).

The five taste receptors on the tongue include sweet, sour, salt, bitter, and the relatively recently cataloged umami, which corresponds to what is sometimes described as the taste of protein, and can be found in miso soup, tomatoes, and fish. The average person has 300,000 taste receptors organized around 6,000 taste buds. The taste buds are found all over the tongue, except at its center. Although it is often claimed that the different receptor types are topographically organized so that different parts of the tongue are dedicated to different taste sensations, it is incorrect, which means that sweet receptors, for example, are not found exclusively on the front part of the tongue.

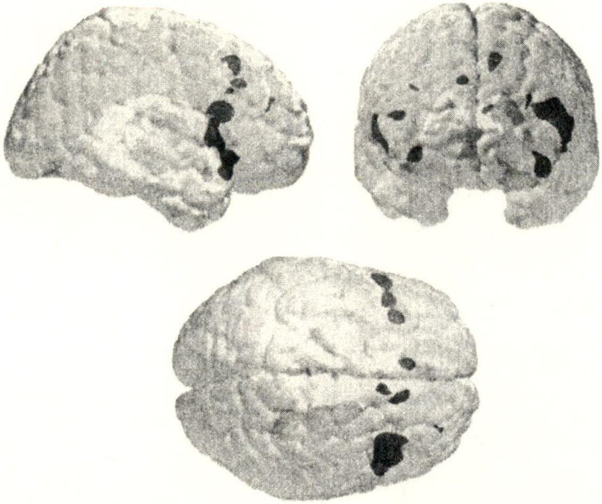

Figure 5.2 Taste. The figure shows a glass brain seen from three different angles (from the side, from the front, and from above) with the primary human taste regions.

Taste information is conveyed from the taste buds to a part of the brainstem (nucleus solitaris) via three large nerve bundles, called the *cranial nerves*. The information is then passed to the thalamus, which receives input from all of the senses except smell, before being conveyed to the primary taste cortex. Scientists have been listening in on the neural activity in this region for monkeys that are given tastants. It turns out that only about 4% to 10% of their neurons react solely to taste. The rest react to other information from the mouth, such as temperature, viscosity, structure, and touch.

Neurons in the primary taste cortex represent the identity of taste, and the patterns of neural activity do not change with how the food is consumed. One can be force-fed without any effect on the neural activity in the primary taste cortex. However, in the secondary taste cortex, force-feeding will lead to changes in the reward value of the sensory input. For example, people will devalue sugar if it is force-fed. These changes in neural responses will often be the first step in a chain of neural activity that will lead to behavioral changes, such as finding ways to stop the force-feeding.

As we chew our food, taste becomes associated with other sensory stimuli, such as smell and touch. Involving these additional senses gives us a better chance to recognize potentially harmful food and save ourselves from becoming ill. Scientists still don't really understand the mechanisms behind how we learn to avoid certain things that are bad for us. They do know that it is a robust kind of learning that goes awry from time to time, as when we develop an aversion to a particular food following an illness—even when the illness is caused by factors other than the food, such as excessive alcohol consumption.

The taste of food causes changes in our brain that enable our digestive system to convert the energy in the food to energy in us. This process relies on the hypothalamus and the striatum. As the link between our reward system and motor behavior, the striatum plays a significant role. A part of the frontal lobes called the *dorsolateral prefrontal cortex* also plays a minor yet interesting role by connecting our decision-making process with our food intake, which is not surprising given that we need to process information to make the decision to take the next bite (Figure 5.3).

Smell

Smell is perhaps the oldest sense and most strongly linked to pleasures and desires. This may be part of the reason that it gives rise to very direct and strong memories, such as those of Proust fame. Another, more prosaic reason might be that, unlike the other senses, smell is not mediated by the main sensory gateway, the thalamus. Our genetic code gives a good indication of how important smell is for us: About 1,000 different genes, corresponding to one of the largest families of genes found in humans, specify our olfactory receptor proteins. Our sense of smell is sophisticated—we can discriminate about half a million unique odors, which may seem staggering until we realize that compared with other mammals, the human sense of smell is not particularly good. The primary olfactory system of dogs, for example, is nearly

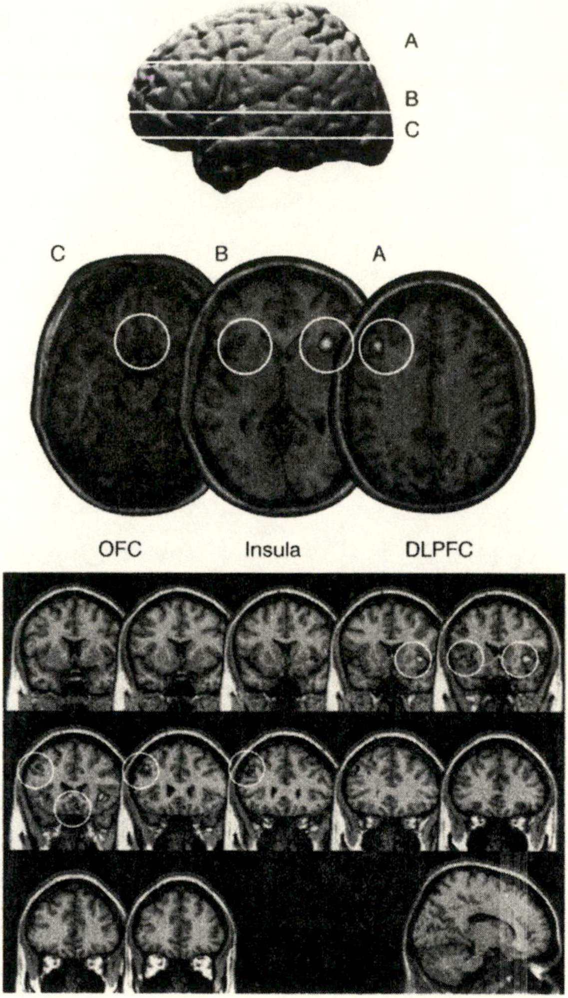

Figure 5.3 More on pure taste in the brain. The figure shows a series of horizontal and vertical slices through the human brain, where there is strongly significant activity related to pure taste. The top panel shows where the horizontal slices are taken. Slice C displays activity in the posterior, medial part of the orbitofrontal cortex, while there is strong bilateral activity in the anterior insular cortex in slice B. Similarly, there is strong taste-related activity in the left dorsolateral prefrontal cortex. At the bottom is shown the spatial extent of this taste-related activity on a series of coronal slices.

three times larger than ours and the olfactory receptors in this space are 100 times more dense than ours.

Our sense of smell begins in the nose, and from there at least five different neural systems bring the sensory inputs to the brain (Figure 5.4). However, smells are not only sensed through our nostrils ("orthonasally") but also through our mouth and throat ("retronasally"). We can perceive the same smell quite differently, depending on which route it takes. With food and drink, the retronasal route is the more important, which is why wine smells different in a glass than in your mouth.

As with the secondary areas for taste, the secondary olfactory areas for smell are more integrative. In them, the olfactory information blends with information from taste and touch. This gives rise to the neural activity corresponding to the crossmodal experience we normally call "taste."

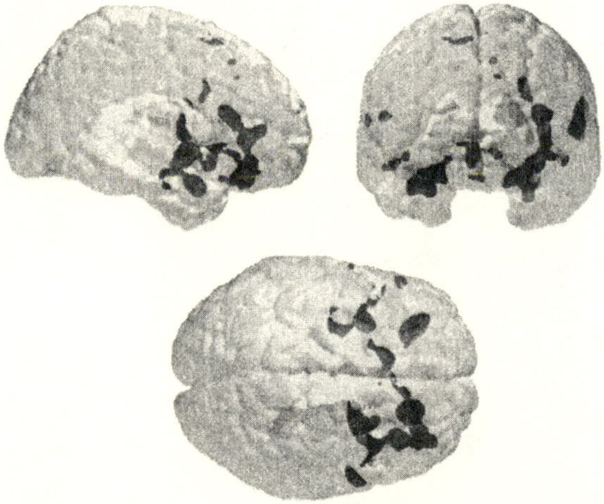

Figure 5.4 Smell. The figure shows a glass brain seen from three different angles (from the side, from the front, and from above) with the primary human olfactory regions.

Scientists have found that a lot of our experience of food and the pleasure we derive from it are represented in different areas of the same brain region, the orbitofrontal cortex: Positive smells, negative smells, the pleasure we derive from smell, and our subjective experience of food are all located in the same brain neighborhood (Figure 5.5).

SMELL, DESIRE, AND REPRODUCTION

When asked which sense is most important to fueling desire and finding a mate, most people would probably say vision, but some research indicates that it is smell. The desires

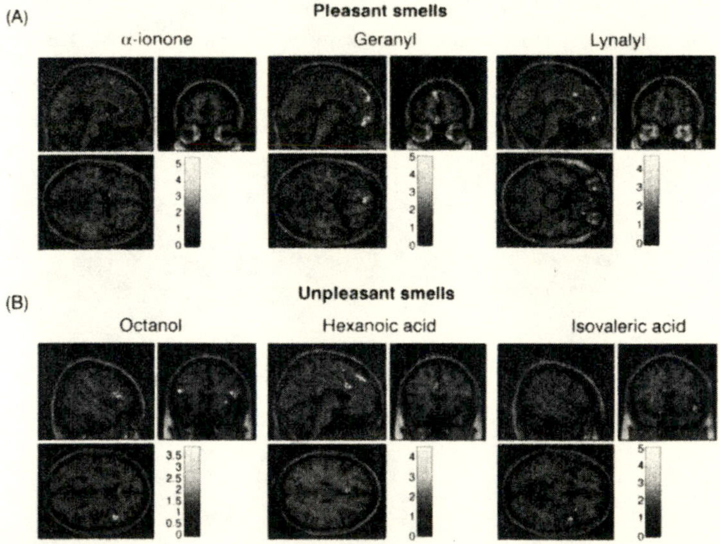

Figure 5.5 More on pure odors. The figure shows the brain activity to three pleasant (A) and unpleasant odors (B). Notice how the pleasant odors give rise to activity in the medial part of the orbitofrontal cortex. The scales show the statistical significance.

brought about by smell are intimately linked to an important olfactory system called *Jacobson's Organ*, which helps to mediate pheromones. Pheromones are airborne chemical substances that can convey information about hormonal balance, and so play an important role in reproduction. Scientists disagree about whether Jacobson's Organ is functional in humans. Some evidence suggests that although the system initially develops in us, just as it does in other animals, it never becomes linked up to the rest of our brain in any functional way. Scientists also disagree about the role of pheromones in human behavior. We know that in animals, pheromones play an important role in regulating behavior, such as when dogs are in heat. But it is not clear whether and to what degree human behavior is also controlled by pheromones, although we do know that they play a role in synchronizing the menstrual cycles of women who live and work together.

Whatever their specific role, it is clear that in humans, pheromones act primarily outside of conscious control and awareness. This means that we're doing a lot of rationalizing after the fact. One interesting example of how these influences may work outside of our conscious awareness is found in some recent experiments involving sweat and T-shirts. A group of men each wore the same T-shirt for 48 hours. Women were then asked to choose a T-shirt by its smell. On average, they chose the T-shirts of men with a different genetic composition than theirs, which is ultimately better for reproduction. Although the women preferred the smell of a different genetic composition, they had no awareness or knowledge of this fact.

Touch

Our sense of touch allows us to get direct physical sensations of the world. In addition to its importance for pleasure and desire, it is also very important for social bonding, which is, in turn, very important for our general emotional stability. Touch is also crucial to how our emotions develop in the first place. Close physical contact between parents and children helps create strong family ties. Orphans deprived of close contact can experience social problems later in life. As detailed in the previous chapter, research on monkeys has very clearly demonstrated the horrible consequences of breaking the bond between mother and infant. Touch is also necessary for food consumption, which we all realize when trying to eat or drink after having had dental work involving Novocain.

The sensations we receive through touch are mediated by sensors on our skin, called *somatosensory receptors*, which have both active and passive components that measure changes in pressure, pain, and temperature. This means that we receive both direct feedback when we are actively investigating the world and indirect feedback even when we aren't carrying out an active investigation. These sensors relay all sensory input information to the brain, which then tries to make sense of the inputs and use them to carry out its second most important job of prediction, trying to predict when and where the next sensory input will arrive. This scenario becomes clear when we investigate why we can't tickle ourselves. Being tickled depends upon not knowing when the next sensory input will arrive. It is all too easy to make these

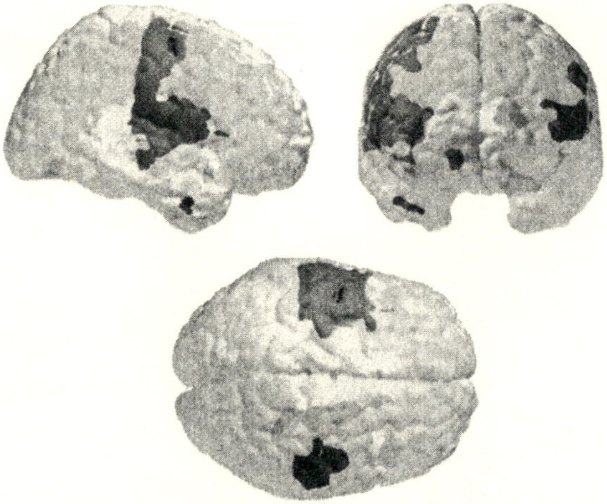

Figure 5.6 Touch. The figure shows a glass brain seen from three different angles (from the side, from the front, and from above) with the primary human somatosensory regions decoding touch to the right hand, which is why the activity is not symmetrical.

predictions for oneself, so it's rather difficult to tickle oneself. If, however, a robotic arm is used that delays and randomly changes its movements, we are easily tickled, even if it is not quite as much fun as being tickled by another person.

The sensory information from the skin receptors flows via the spinal cord to the primary somatosensory cortex, where the whole surface of the body is represented in a number of maps (Figure 5.6).

These brain maps are proportional to density of the receptors on the skin, rather than to the actual surface of our body, so their representation of our body is disproportional and skewed. This inaccurate representation reveals some interesting facts about the importance of certain body parts that serve to sustain us: the genitals, the face, and the

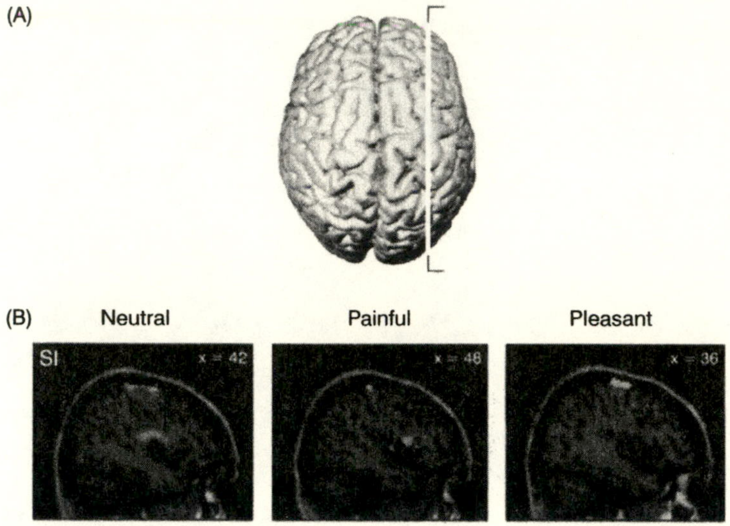

Figure 5.7 More on affective touch. (A) shows where the slices in (B) are taken in the brain. Neutral, painful, and pleasant touch to the right hand evoke activity in the same part of primary somatosensory cortex.

mouth. The face and the genitals occupy a disproportional larger area in the brain than the elbow and the toes. The map of the face is not next to the one of the neck, but of the hand, and the map of the genitals is not next to that of the legs, but of the feet. The sensory maps for the mouth are extensive, as assessing food requires precise sensory information about whether it has the right texture, which is clear when you notice how different the same food tastes when only the texture is different, as when it is wet and dry (Figure 5.7).

Vision

Vision is the sensory system that takes up the most space in the human brain, and probably the one that has contributed most to the survival of our species, as it allows us to avoid danger by detecting threats at a distance. It should not be surprising, then, that by some estimates almost half of the human brain is dedicated to processing the various aspects of visual stimuli. Vision is also an excellent example of how little insight we have into the functioning of our brain, as the majority of its very complicated processing is nonconscious. When we look around, we see everything in focus all the time. This is an amazingly powerful illusion, given that we have a blind spot in each eye and a visual angle such that fewer than two degrees of our retina are in focus at any one time (Figure 5.8).

Most of us also are not aware that our eyes make nearly imperceptible movements four times per second. These movements are called *saccades* and help maintain the illusion that the full visual field is in focus. But saccades also have other functions. When people are looking at faces, the saccades follow the shape of the face in nearly the same way as blind people become familiar with a face by touching it (Figure 5.9). The idea that seeing is like touching at a distance can be traced back to the eighteenth century writings of the English philosopher George Berkeley; this idea was recently resurrected by the English brain scientist Rodney Cotterill. Vision may indeed at times work a bit like the sense of touch, but usually at a safe distance, as its main evolutionary function has been to allow us to react quickly if, for example, a lion jumps in our path.

Visual processing starts when light falls on the retina. The main sensory receptors, rods and cones, convert light to nerve signals that flow from the eyes through the thalamus

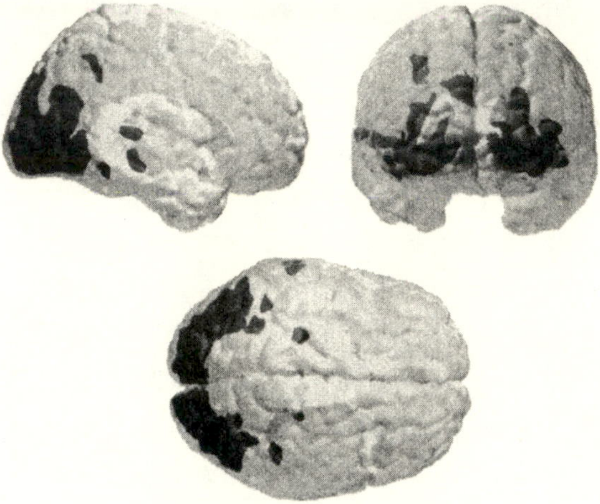

Figure 5.8 Vision. The figure shows a glass brain seen from three different angles (from the side, from the front, and from above) with the primary human visual regions.

to the primary visual cortex at the back of the brain. The visual impressions are upside down in the primary visual cortices, making the images processed by the brain both mirrored and inverted from its form in the sensory world. Visual impressions then make their way back to the front of the brain along two more or less separate pathways, corresponding to the "what" and the "where" of the visual scene. Along the way, these impressions pass through a hierarchy of areas, each of which corresponds to a specialized type of processing, such as those for form, color, and movement. As with the processing for the other senses, the information is maintained separately at first, but then integrated as it is processed in higher-order visual areas. There has, however, been substantial debate over whether object processing is in fact localized to certain regions or distributed over many

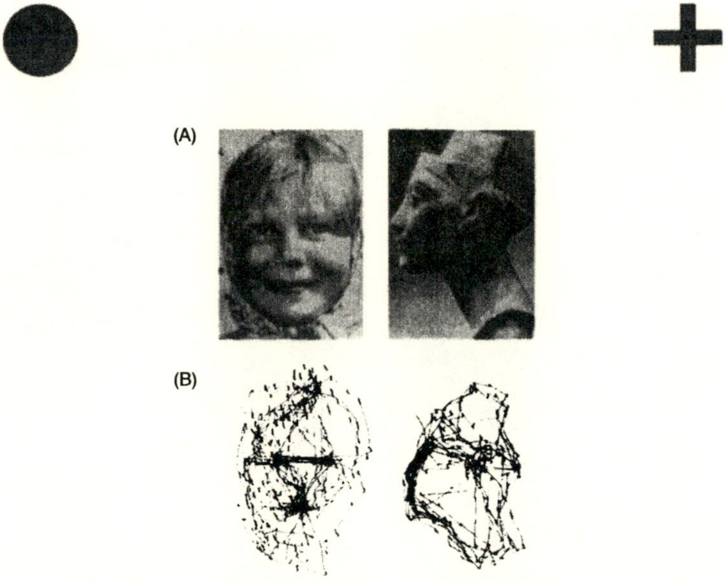

Figure 5.9 The blind spot and saccadic eye movements. (A) allows you to find the blind spot in your eye. Close your right eye and focus your left eye on the cross, while moving the book around 12 inches from your eye. This will make the big dot disappear. It is a good example of how the brain spontaneously invents a plausible story about missing information. (B) shows the saccadic eye movements made over approximately 2 minutes. It is interesting to note how these eye movements track the contours; remarkably like touching objects at a distance.

regions in the cortex, so it is important to note that the scientific jury is still out on the amount of functional specificity in vision.

Hearing

If we are unable to see the lion because it is hiding behind a bush, waiting for an appropriate snack, our sense of hearing can be rather helpful. The main function of hearing, however, is its pivotal role in mediating our pleasures and desires. Hearing is particularly crucial for decoding human language and music (Figure 5.10).

Our sense of hearing depends on being able to capture sounds through receptors in various structures of our inner ear. Sounds are waves in the air that are channeled by the outer ear to the eardrum. These waves create vibrations in the inner ear that are carried by an ingenious mechanical system to the oval window and the cochlea. The cochlea is filled with 16,000 hair cells that react differently, depending on the frequency of the vibration. These hair cells connect with neurons in the brainstem and send the sound signals via the thalamus to the primary and then the secondary auditory cortices, where they are analyzed in detail.

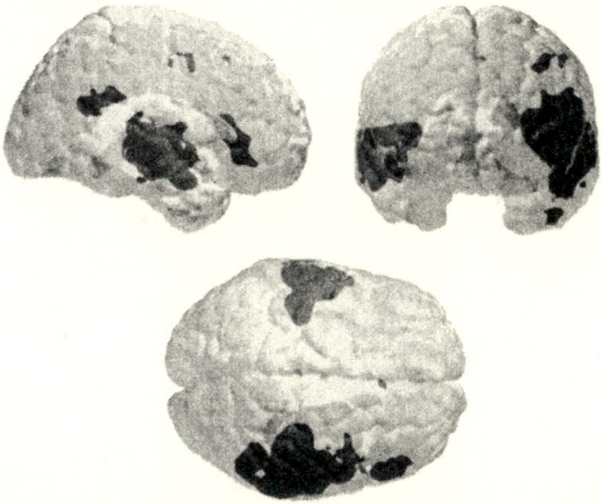

Figure 5.10 Hearing. The figure shows a glass brain seen from three different angles (from the side, from the front, and from above) with the primary human auditory regions.

As we saw with taste, different qualities, such as viscosity and elasticity, must be analyzed separately. In hearing, it is most important to distinguish between the intensity and frequency of sounds. In the primary auditory cortex, different groups of neurons react only to tones within a certain frequency. The position of the sound relative to the body is also important, and our brains determine this position by analyzing the relative delay of the sound from one ear to another.

● LEAVING OUR SENSES

In the following chapters, we will see how the brain uses this sensory information to create complex representations of the world, which allows us not only to survive and reproduce but also to have unique subjective experiences.

● ● ● HAPPINESS LESSON

Our senses offer primal delights, especially where food is concerned. Enjoy those delights, in moderation, and seek variation.

The fundamental pleasures

The fundamental pleasures are elicited by the sensations involved in food intake, sex, and social interactions. The sensations are detected by sensory receptors which are then decoded in the primary sensory regions in the brain. Pleasure is not a sensation, but linked to the anticipation, evaluation, and memory of sensations. Research in humans and other animals has shown that certain networks of brain regions and neurotransmitters are essential to pleasure. Some of these regions are found deep in the brain (nucleus accumbens, ventral pallidum, amygdala, periaqueductal grey, hypothalamus, ventral tegmental area) and others in the cortex (orbitofrontal, cingulate and insular cortices). Higher order pleasures have been shown to reuse the same pleasure networks as the fundamental pleasures.

FURTHER READING

The senses in the brain have been explored for many years, but new and surprising findings take time to make it into books. My students have found the following books most helpful:

Bear, M. F., Connors, B. W. & Paradiso, M. A. (2006). *Neuroscience. Exploring the Brain.* 3rd ed, New York, NY: Lippincott, Williams & Wilkins.

Gazzaniga, M. (2004). *The New Cognitive Neurosciences.* 3rd ed., Cambridge, MA: MIT Press.

Kandel, E., Schwartz, J. & Jessell, T. (2000). *Principles of Neural Science.* 4th ed., New York, NY: McGraw-Hill.

6

MEMORIES

To Forget is to Remember

...to think is to forget a difference, to generalize, to abstract.

J.L. Borges (1899–1986)

In the beginning of the twentieth century, a young woman was hospitalized with such pervasive memory loss as a result of serious brain damage that the staff and her doctor had to reintroduce themselves every time. Slightly annoyed by this, Dr. Edouard Claparède set out to find out whether the young woman really had completely forgotten. Rather mischievously, he hid a pin in his hand the next time he reintroduced himself by offering a handshake. Claparède then left the room and came back a while later. The young woman was still unable to recognize him, but she refused to shake hands from then on. She was unable to explain why, but she was apparently able to remember without being conscious of being able to remember. This case demonstrates how the brain's hedonic evaluations may proceed nonconsciously and come to shape our behavior without us knowing why.

Most of us are luckily spared the devastating experience of amnesia following brain damage, yet we are all prone to peculiar lapses of memory and reason. This was demonstrated by a simple, yet elegant experiment led recently by Swedish philosopher Lars Hall. In the experiment, participants were shown pairs of cards with photos of young women on them and given as much time as they would like to choose the more attractive one. The cards would then be laid face down and the participant would be given the card they had chosen. Participants would explain at some length why they chose this woman. What the participants did not know was that the experimenter was a trained magician who would from time to time swap the cards around and instead give the participant the card they had just rejected. Most of the participants did not notice this swap, but continued to happily confabulate about why they had chosen the card they had in fact just rejected.

How do such reevaluations of our hedonic evaluations come about? We are prone to start to report pleasurable memories of situations that were far from pleasurable at the time. The struggles against great adversity, such as acts of resistance during wartime, are often recollected as happy memories of a time where we did not in fact experience much pleasure.

Brain research is still struggling to understand the many faces of memory. It has become increasingly clear that memory is not a unitary concept, but that the brain stores information in many different ways. Memory and learning are closely linked and it is difficult to see how learning can occur without ways of storing what has been learned. As with so much other activity in the brain, we are only conscious of a small part of these brain processes. In fact, sometimes it would appear that we have so little insight into our own memory that this leads us to confabulate. As we shall see in the following topics, perhaps the most paradoxical recent scientific insight is that we get better at remembering by forgetting.

THE ANATOMY OF OBLIVION

A 30-year-old man came to see the Russian neuroscientist Alexander Romanovitch Luria in the early 1920s. The man, Solomon Shereshevsky, had tried to become a musician, but had settled for journalism. When the journalists at the newspaper where he worked convened in the morning to discuss the program of the day, all except Shereshevsky brought out their pads to take down the details. Shereshevsky habitually put pen to paper only when the final article had to go to press. The editor voiced his concern on several occasions, but Shereshevsky never forgot even the smallest detail. Indeed, detail characterized his writing to the extent that extraneous details crept in everywhere.

As time went on, this amount of detail became too much for the editor and he decided to have Shereshevsky tested by a psychologist. At the time, Dr. Luria was still a young man, and had yet to make his reputation as one the most important psychologists of the twentieth century. This reputation partly rests on his thorough investigations of the apparently inexhaustible memory of the person known as S., who was of course none other than the journalist Shereshevsky.

To test the limits of Shereshevsky's memory, Luria would read out long sequences of numbers and words, which Shereshevsky subsequently repeated without error, not only from the beginning, but also backward. It did not seem to matter whether the words had meaning or how many elements he was asked to remember. But even more remarkable was the durability of his memory. When Luria eventually tested him on sequences memorized 15 years earlier, Shereshevsky consistently recalled them without error.

The amazing memory of Shereshevsky was not the result of tricks such as those often employed by professional mnemonists. Such people will memorize, for example, the Koran or London's A to Z. Although remarkable as expressions of sheer willpower, such feats lack the effortlessness of Shereshevsky's memory because they require huge amounts of concentration and constant exercise. Given the right training, almost everyone is able to learn their mnemonic techniques of encoding information as a visual narrative. They include a simple method of committing to memory each element by tying them to landmarks on a well-known walk. To recall the information, one mentally rehearses the walk and the elements are recalled as they occur during the mental walk. The senators in ancient Rome were known to use this oratory trick by mentally linking information to the pillars of the Senate.

The Struggle to Forget

Shereshevsky did not appear to use any conscious strategy for encoding and recalling information. Memories accumulated partly against his will, so it was forgetting that required his concentration. When he heard a story, he would spontaneously form vivid mental images, which later helped him to recall the story accurately. But these mental images also made it hard for him to understand the essence of even simple stories. For instance if he heard a story of a merchant, he would immediately imagine the merchant in his shop with a plethora of irrelevant details. He might imagine the arrival of a customer, and then suddenly, notice the writing in account books or other irrelevant details, thus disrupting the storyline.

These irrelevant details would almost overwhelm Shereshevsky and hinder his understanding of the essential facts. When he started working as a professional mnemonist, these problems became ever more taxing. Often he performed in the same place and with the same blackboard containing long sequences of random letters, numbers, and words that he had to remember. In order not to confound his different performances, Shereshevsky would imagine that the blackboard was covered with an impenetrable film that could be crumpled and thrown away later. However, even when using this odd mental technique, sequences from earlier performances would still sometimes blend with the current performance, so he occasionally would appear to misremember.

To solve this problem, Shereshevsky thought that just as some people write down what they want to remember, he could write down the things he wanted to forget. He hoped that if he wrote something down, he no longer would need to remember it. Unfortunately, and perhaps not surprisingly, this not only failed to solve his problem, it aggravated it. In desperation, he tried to burn his notes. This was no better because he could still read the notes on the burning ember. As time passed, his inability to forget became an almost unbearable torment.

Finally, just as he had almost given up hope of ever being able to forget, he suddenly found a simple, if almost banal, way to solve the problem. All he had to do was to consciously *decide* to forget, and the memories would fade. Brain-scanning techniques had not been invented during Shereshevsky's lifetime, so we do not know whether his brain was different from that of other people, exactly how his extraordinary memory worked, and why for so long he was seemingly unable to forget.

BLENDING OF THE SENSES

Closely linked to Shereshevsky's extraordinary memory was another phenomenon: When Shereshevsky heard a sound, it would immediately trigger other sensory experiences of light, touch, color, and taste. Different sensory impressions would instantly blend with each other. For him, the phoneme *a* was "something white and long," while the number 8 had "a naïve quality, it is milky blue like lime." This blending of sensory qualities is called *synesthesia*. Many people will experience a mild degree of synesthesia, such as when vowels and consonants evoke different colors or a given tone is experienced as "warm" or "cold." But synesthesia is rarely found to such an extreme degree as it was found in Shereshevsky.

Synesthesia provided Shereshevsky with the intensity of deeply personal experiences and conveyed extra information that let him correctly recall even the most insignificant details. On the rare occasions when he remembered imperfectly, synesthesia provided the sensory qualities that acted as an error-correction mechanism and allowed him to correct the mistake.

What was most interesting about Shereshevsky were the general principles that could be extracted from his case. The phenomenal always carries the universal within it. Some people may have photographic—*eidetic*—memories in early childhood only to lose this ability in puberty. We have yet to discover the reason, but some scientific evidence suggests that it is linked with the development of the brain structures in the prefrontal cortex. We are still preoccupied by the puzzles raised by Shereshevsky's case. A key may lie in a better understanding of synesthesia, and brain scanning of synesthetes is starting to add knowledge.

SYNESTHESIA

Synesthesia came into the English language in 1891 from the Greek words for blending, *syn,* and senses, *aisthesis.* However, the phenomenon was known long before, in 1690, with one of the first written accounts from the English philosopher John Locke. Francis Galton described synesthesia from a more scientific viewpoint in 1880. As with much of Galton's research (which included some dubious eugenic speculations), there have been divided and often strong opinions about its significance. Many people wrote off synesthesia as a side effect of drug abuse, given that hallucinogenic drugs such as LSD can give rise to similar sensory blending in the hinterland between hallucinations and reality. Yet only a small percentage of people have regular use of such drugs, so such explanations seem unlikely. Nevertheless, it was only recently that scientists started to seriously study synesthesia using brain-scanning techniques.

A common explanation of synesthesia is based on association learning in early childhood. One argument is that some synesthetes may have played with types of toys that let them form close memories and associations between the sensory aspects of these toys. For instance, the toy letters may have different colors that are later reproduced. However, this does not explain why only some people have these strong sense-blending experiences.

It would seem obvious to ask synesthetes how they experience the sensory blending. But very few are certain of whether they experience the blending directly or from memory. So we're forced to trust that they really experience the sensory blending. Fortunately, however, it is possible to test the level of synesthesia. One technique takes its inspiration from pop-out figures, such as those used to test for color blindness. Based only on their colors, a number of similar shapes can be made to form different simple patterns. People who are color blind are unable to see certain colors, so they are also unable to see these patterns, which are easily seen by people with normal color vision.

A similar principle is used in testing for synesthesia. Shapes such as 2 and 5 can be made to look very similar to normal people, while synesthetes experience special colors and get a much quicker pop-out effect.

However, such visual techniques obviously are not appropriate for blind synesthetes who experience color percepts for certain kinds of words. Instead one has to ascertain consistency over time in the sensory qualities experienced.

We investigated a middle-aged blind man who reported experiencing colors when he heard words related to time. He became blind very early in life. Using various brain-scanning techniques, we found activity in the part of visual cortex that is related to color processing in sighted people. This color-related activity was specific to time even in synonyms: For example, when he heard the word "March," he experienced colors only when the word was used as the month, not as a verb meaning to walk.

So the balance of the evidence shows that synesthesia is a real phenomenon that is found in more than 1 in 2000 people. Through systematic neuroimaging investigations of synesthesia, we now know how and where sensory blending occurs in the brain. Because synesthesia is reported as the experience of sensory blending, one possible explanation for the phenomenon might be mixed-up connections between the different sensory regions. This fits with Chapter 5, showing how visual stimuli are processed in ever greater detail through hierarchical networks stretching from the back to the front of the brain.

Similar principles of gradual processing take place for the other senses, so synesthesia could come about through excessive connections between the senses early on in the cortical processing stream. While this certainly is an attractive hypothesis, it is also now clear that this is unlikely to be the full explanation. It is also unlikely that synesthesia in itself is the key to Shereshevsky's formidable memory, since most synesthetes do not have anything comparable to his *eidetic* abilities.

TO FORGET IS TO REMEMBER

Using experimental animals and brain scanning, science has come closer to an understanding of memory. In particular, it has become clear that memory is not a unitary phenomenon, but consists of many subsystems and mechanisms. A brain without memory is not particularly useful because all learning relies on the ability to store information to learn from mistakes. The study of memory may eventually help us decipher some of the functions of the brain.

This potential can be illustrated with an example. Focus on the following words, try to remember them, and then read on, candy, sour, sugar, good, taste, tooth, delicious, honey, soft drink, chocolate, heart, cake, eat, tart.

Without looking at the words again, try to remember whether the words *taste, point,* and *sweet* were on the list. Most people are certain that the word *sweet* is on the list, although it is not. It is a simple example of how memory can mislead.

A first attempt at understanding how memory can mislead is to note all the taste-related words on the list. Most of us easily remember that *taste* is on the list and that *point* is not. But *sweet* is different, given that it is clearly related to taste. The presence of related words such as *sugar, chocolate,* and *soft drink* may make us think that *sweet* is, present too. But this cannot be the full explanation, as shown in the following.

CONSCIOUS REMEMBERING

The example of taste-related words shows how the conscious act of remembering depends on how the brain first encodes information and then recalls this memory. Encoding and recall are therefore dual aspects of the act of remembering. A good example of this dual aspect is the sentence "The fish attacked the swimmer." Most people erroneously come to recall that it was a shark that attacked the swimmer, and are more likely to recall the sentence if given a prime of *shark* rather than *fish*.

The example shows how we first process a sentence semantically by using our knowledge of sharks and fish before we encode the memory. Experiments on amnesiacs, patients with severe memory problems, have shown that because some are unable to use this semantic preprocessing, they are not distracted by the difference between fish and sharks and thus they are able to remember the sentence more accurately than normal people are.

Our conscious recall also functions over different time spans. Fundamentally, there are clear differences between short- and long-term memory. Experiments have shown that short-term memory in normal people probably is limited to seven—"plus or minus two"—memory items. The example with fifteen mostly taste-related words also exceeds the limit on our short-term memory systems. Because we find it hard to remember them all, we try to encode them according to meaning and transfer them to long-term memory, which, other scientific experiments have shown, is practically unlimited but rarely perfect.

The conscious transfer of memories from short- to long-term memory appears to be carried out in the cortex in the temporal lobes. Historically, much effort has been devoted to understanding the functions of the *hippocampus*, a structure deep in the temporal lobes, which was given its Latin name for its apparent likeness to a seahorse.

This structure is often damaged in amnesiacs. The classic example of hippocampal damage is that of patient HM, who was treated for severe epilepsy by removal of large parts of the temporal lobes including the hippocampus and the amygdala. After his operation, HM was unable to learn new names or remember events that occurred since his operation. But he still was able to remember events that occurred before it.

Researchers have since tried to repeat these experiments on monkeys with precise lesions of the hippocampus, but without great success. Studies in other human patients with more precise lesions to the hippocampus have shown that the hippocampal damage is unlikely to be the root of HM's memory problems. Instead, it is clear that the cortex just below the hippocampus in the entorhinal and perirhinal cortex appear to be essential for the correct transfer or consolidation from short- to long-term memory.

The hippocampus is probably mostly related to spatial memories, as shown by studying rats that have had it removed. They were unable to remember where a platform is hidden in a water basin filled with milky water (in the so-called "Morris water maze" named after the Scottish neuroscientist John Morris). Other experiments from the beginning of the 1970s by the English neurophysiologist

John O'Keefe and colleagues show that the hippocampus appears to store maps of the environment. The researchers recorded the neural activity in the hippocampus of rats and found maps in which some neurons responded maximally when the rat was in a certain location with a reward. Similar maps have not been found in the hippocampus of humans or monkeys, which may relate to the difference in anatomy between rats and higher primates. Unlike rats, which move on four legs and whose head movement appears to have less freedom, primates appear to have hippocampal cells that store information about the position of the head in relation to the body and to the environment.

UNCONSCIOUS MEMORIES

It has been shown that amnesiacs who are incapable of conscious recollection are in fact capable of new learning. However, they remain unaware of this. Research over the last couple of years has given greater insights into the mechanisms of unconscious memory. This type of memory is typically called *procedural* or *implicit memory* and is linked to the learning of skills and the development of habits. This is in contrast to the conscious recollections typically called *semantic* or *explicit memory*, which are linked to factual, semantic, and conceptual knowledge.

Implicit memory can be demonstrated in priming experiments in which a couple of words are shown for such brief intervals that the participants remain unaware of them. But showing a partial word such as "*c***o**te*" makes the participants much better on average at recognizing the partial word as one of the subsequent primes, "chocolate." This is also true for amnesiacs, who can thus be shown to be able to remember without being able to remember. Similarly, they can gain new motor skills, such as playing the piano without having conscious recollections of ever having done so.

Some evidence points to the amygdala as an important structure in the formation of implicit memories, especially those with an emotional content. This may be linked to why Claparède's patient was able to remember that she did not like handshakes without remembering why. Her conscious memory systems had become damaged, but the nonconscious system was still functioning.

But how do these conscious memory systems work? In order to be stored, a memory must become consolidated. That means it must be able to transfer from short- to long-term memory and to show resistance to brain damage. Examples of such resistance can be seen in patients with anterograde amnesia, who have trouble remembering anything after the accident, but who can remember events before the accident. Most patients with retrograde amnesia have trouble remembering recent events before the accident, including the accident itself, although they remember events from a more distant past.

Memories become robust through becoming distributed in the brain. Take for example how the memories of an orange are stored in the brain. Recollection of an orange involves a process in which all of these sensory qualities—its orange color, round shape, granulated surface, and acid taste—are reconstructed to the memory of an orange. This recall process is like a giant puzzle that is put together on the fly from the prompt of just a few pieces.

Therefore, damage to the brain regions representing visual color can lead to the loss of ability not only to see color but also to *recall* it. Fortunately, the brain exhibits excellent plasticity, meaning that some regions can replace the functionality of other regions. The precise mechanisms for consolidation are still unknown and appear to involve the amygdala and the reactivation of a memory. Some researchers have proposed that sleep and dreaming play a central role in the consolidation processes, but this remains speculative.

CONFABULATIONS AND CREATIVE DISTORTIONS

While most patients with memory problems have suffered damage to their temporal lobes, some amnesic patients have instead suffered damage to their medial orbitofrontal cortex. These patients are much more prone to invent narratives that are not consistent with reality. Evidence from the card experiment (mentioned in the beginning of the chapter) and other experiments appear to suggest that we all share this propensity to invent narratives.

So, to remember is a creative process; rather than saying that we *remember* an event, perhaps we should say that we *recreate* the event. Evidence from criminal cases has shown that memories are easily distorted. The word-list example earlier showed the same. (Can you still remember the elements on the list?) We seldom recount a story in exactly the same way each time, and the story often changes from when we first heard it. This encoding process can change the information in important ways, as we saw in the shark example in which we used our preexisting knowledge for the erroneous consolidation.

Distortion of memories is therefore a natural property of our memory systems. Memories are stored over large regions of the brain as patterns of activity upon earlier patterns. This means that our memories are not exact copies of an event, but dependent on our personal history. More exactly, because memory is not a carbon copy of events forgetting becomes a necessary function of memory.

We are often left with a sense of the emotion attached to the memories. But even this can become distorted, reinterpreted and changed in the light of our personal history. We speak of character building as an important element of life-changing events, and although most of these events often felt quite painful when they occurred, with time we are likely to change our recollection of them.

This means that the attempts to improve our memory by chemical means also have to help with forgetting. There has been much discussion in the pharmaceutical industry about the prospect of creating a pill that can bolster failing memories. Some of this enthusiasm stems from Nobel Prize–winning research by Austrian-American psychiatrist Eric Kandel and his colleagues to understand the underlying memory principles in the Aplysia snail. The commercial exploitation of the molecular and biochemical insights from this research has been underway for some time now. As yet, a memory pill has yet to emerge. Some researchers remain skeptical about whether it is possible to slow the natural aging properties of memory without introducing other problems.

All the same, some researchers are hopeful that we may be able to alleviate the symptoms for people with Alzheimer's disease, first described by the German neuropathologist Alois Alzheimer in 1906. Everyone who has experienced losing a close family member or friend to this progressive disease knows how the disease slowly removes the traces of the person that once was.

Memory is closely tied to what it means to be human and even if our understanding of the memory mechanisms in the brain is greater than ever before, we are still far from a full understanding. We have made significant progress in understanding the brain mechanisms and molecular principles of memory. In particular, we have improved our understanding of how learning and memory interact, but we will return to this theme in later chapters.

● ● ● HAPPINESS LESSONS

Just because you can't remember something consciously doesn't mean you don't remember it at all. If you "have a feeling" about something, there may be a very good reason behind that feeling. That is, trust your intuitions. On the other hand, beware of unwarranted assumptions.

If you want to remember something, reinforce that memory: attach emotional significance and link to existing visual landmarks, for example, a specific walk.

FURTHER READING

Although the puzzles of memory are still unsolved, there is a long list of excellent books on the subject. Luria's monograph on Shereshevsky is a modern classic: Luria, A. R. (1968) *The Mind of a Mnemonist: A Little Book about a Vast Memory.* Harvard University Press, Cambridge, Mass.

Borges' story about Funes' similar problems with memory is even more readable: Borges, J. L. (1944) *Ficciones.* Weidenfeld, New York.

Of more recent brain oriented books on memory the following are excellent examples: Schacter, D. L. (1999) *Searching for memory. The brain, the mind and the past.* Basic Books, New York. Squire, L. R. & E.R., K. (1999) *Memory: From Mind to Molecules.* W.H. Freeman & Co., New York.

7

LEARNING

Emotions and Thoughts

> Education is an admirable thing, but it is well to remember from time to time that nothing that is worth knowing can be taught.
>
> Oscar Wilde (1854–1900)

When I was a young boy, my grandfather took me for long walks on the beach. Among the pebbles at the edge of the ocean were many fossils, including thunderstones. These are fossils of extinct animals in the squid family that lived in the Jurassic and Cretaceous periods. They can be difficult to discern among the pebbles, so it requires training and concentration to find them. They are sufficiently common along Danish beaches so that, unlike the less common amber, they hold no monetary value. Nevertheless, I desired them for their long semitransparent golden shape and for the pleasure of the hunt. My grandfather was an expert in finding thunderstones and one of my greatest ambitions was to become as skilled.

Learning is commonly associated with lessons and classrooms. But Oscar Wilde was right to point out that nothing that is worth knowing can be taught. Collecting thunderstones is not a subject in any school I know of. To learn it, I needed only plenty of time and motivation, which are some of the most important elements for learning. Other ones include a certain amount of talent and a good portion of luck.

Desire and pleasure are central for learning. They are involved in the possible causes for poor mathematical abilities, stuttering, and dyslexia. They underlie the brain mechanisms that form the basis of the insights, creativity, and thinking which are closely linked to good, effective learning.

THE NUMBER SENSE

Unlike thunderstone collecting, mathematical abilities are commonly described as desirable, especially among employers. Nevertheless, many people happily claim that they are hopeless at math. Some will even go as far as to claim that they were born without any mathematical sense, and that no amount of motivation would make a difference. However, research shows that children and even other animals have a natural aptitude for numbers, and both number sense and mathematics can be learned.

One of the most well-known examples of what might appear as the product of innate mathematical ability came about in the beginning of the last century. In 1913, the

English Cambridge professor of mathematics G.H. Hardy received a letter from what was then known as Madras, India. The letter, sent by a young Indian man named Srinavasa Ramanujan Iyengar, was written in a style that almost made Hardy throw away the letter. But a series of long mathematical formulas toward the end of the letter was to change the destiny of both Hardy and mathematics.

The complex, slightly strange mathematical formulas in the letter consisted partly of a series of well-known theorems, some of which were derived in roundabout ways from deep mathematical results that Hardy had contributed to. The other part consisted of a string of apparently obscure formulas using long lists of square roots, exponentials, and fractions. As Hardy worked with ever greater enthusiasm through the formulas, he realized that the letter had to be the work of a mathematical genius.

Ramanujan was hurriedly summoned to Cambridge; until his tragic death in 1929, he contributed a wide range of mathematical theorems and proofs. But he had received only 9 years of schooling, without any particular mathematical training. He had never been to university, but through careful study of books had developed his amazing skills. Was Ramanujan a unique genius, or do we all carry the possibility of becoming like him?

RETARDED GENIUS

In some ways, Michael has a mathematical talent like that of Ramanujan, yet in the most important ways, it is different. Michael is autistic and has never learned to talk. He shows no signs of being able to understand words, so he cannot be tested on a verbal intelligence quotient (IQ) test. His nonverbal IQ has been measured at 67, which is significantly below the average IQ score of 100.

But Michael possesses formidable arithmetical abilities. Since the age of 6, he has been fascinated by pure numbers, money, clocks, calendars, and maps. On logical IQ tests, he scores 128, which is well above average. Michael cannot name objects, but needs just over a second to decide whether a given three-digit number is a prime. How can Michael be unable to speak and mentally backward, but lightning quick at mental arithmetic?

As Ramanujan lay dying of tuberculosis, Hardy was a frequent visitor. One day Hardy remarked that his taxi was numbered 1729, which seemed to him a dull number. Ramanujan promptly replied that, in his opinion, this was far from the case because it is the smallest number that can be described in two different ways as the sum of the cube of two numbers.

Most people find somewhat odd both the idea of calculating the cube of a number and having an intuitive understanding that the number 1729 is special. But many people find it easy to talk for hours about the various plants in their garden. Perhaps some mathematicians are just as knowledgeable about numbers as amateur gardeners are about the contents of their garden. Some may even have extensive knowledge of both. My oldest daughter is convinced that one of our eminent mathematicians at The Queen's College is in fact the resident gardener in what she regards as her own magical college garden.

An example of another gardener of numbers is the French mathematician François Le Lionnais, who published the fruits of his lifelong fascination with numbers in 1983. His book *Nombres Remarquables* is filled with many remarkable numbers and their special attributes. For example, the number 39 is the smallest natural number that does not have any special attributes (which of course raises the question of whether this number should be included in a book of remarkable numbers).

Perhaps the comparison between number sense and gardens is not half bad. It has been shown that children who are good at solving spatial tasks in general are comparably better at mathematics. This result has also received some backing from brain-scanning experiments that have shown that neighboring regions of the parietal cortices are used for spatial representations and calculations.

GENDER HYGIENE

In most Western societies, mathematical ability is a sure admission ticket to a higher education. The implicit belief is that those with mathematical abilities are more intelligent than those without. Some researchers claim to have shown that men generally are better than women at mathematical tests. Some researchers have used this sex difference to claim that this is the natural order of society. These researchers are also prone to attach great significance to the alleged racial differences in intelligence discussed in an earlier chapter. In other words, the status quo of a male-dominated society is only the consequence of the supposed fact that women are more stupid than men.

At this point, it is hoped that such assertions seem unfounded and unhelpful, but still they point to a fundamental problem in education. Many psychological and sociological factors conspire to make it harder for women to succeed in mathematics. Professional mathematicians are almost exclusively men, and most women find mathematics too remote from the real world to occupy them. Women therefore tend to become better gardeners—or whatever they take pleasure in—than mathematicians. However, most countries value mathematics more highly than gardening skills, which affects access to education. Many of those without mathematical insight are all too easily deprived of those educational opportunities that could have made a significant difference in their lives.

It may seem strange that mathematics has gained priority over other equally important mental abilities of our social brains, such as compassion and empathy. The standard answer is that mathematics has been instrumental in the technological feats of humanity, which are central to our standards of living and to societal structures in general. So it may be unrealistic to expect much change in educational politics.

But it is clear that everyone can learn number manipulation and even advanced mathematics. Experiments on babies have shown how the ability to handle numbers is a part of our basic mental equipment. Well-controlled experiments in monkeys and other animals have shown that some animals also have a fundamental understanding of numbers. Rosenkrantz and MacDuff are rhesus monkeys studied by the American neuroscientists Elizabeth M. Brannon and

Herbert S. Terrace at Columbia University, New York. The monkeys have astounded the scientific community by being able to arrange numerical sets in the correct order.

The monkeys are shown up to nine objects on a computer screen. The task is to touch the images in numerical order as we would arrange a deck of cards according to value. The monkeys *numerate*, which is an ability that is closely related to having a number sense. The researchers also have recorded neural activity in the monkeys' brains and shown that some neurons show activity that correlates with the size of the numbers. Similar findings of neural activity correlated with the size of numbers also have been shown in neuroimaging experiments in humans.

This evidence also fits well with the poor understanding of numbers that is shown by patients who have suffered damage to specific parts of the brain. For example, Noam is unable to carry out precise calculations. When asked to calculate the result of "two plus two," he answers "three." So it would seem likely that he has completely lost his mathematical abilities. But it turns out that he has some other basic number skills, which include knowing that eight is larger than seven and that 75 is closer to 100 than to 10. His mathematical abilities are like those of Rosenkrantz and MacDuff, because Noam has kept his fundamental quantitative abilities, but has lost his abstract manipulation skills.

MATHEMATICAL GARDENING

So the balance of the scientific evidence would seem to indicate that both humans and other animals are imbued with a natural capacity for mathematics. Although Ramanujan had no formal education, he was highly motivated, which is important for a talent to be nurtured and developed. He also was lucky, in that Hardy was ready to bring him to England. Hardy then added the necessary discipline to trim and complement Ramanujan's extraordinary mathematical intuition.

Michael and Ramanujan are not so very different in their obsession with numbers. But Ramanujan appears to have achieved a better balance with those other abilities that Michael is clearly missing. On the other hand, despite motivation, it will remain very difficult for Noam to learn to carry out precise calculations because of his brain damage.

Starting with Galileo, some people have stated that the universe is written in the language of mathematics. The evidence so far from neuroscience shows that our brains are not logical, universal, or optimal. Our brains may be reasonably good with numbers, but remain poor at logic and complex calculations. So although mathematics may be the language of the universe, it is more likely to remain a tool with which our brains can try to read the structure of the universe.

But given that most tasks and jobs in this world are not about understanding the structure of the universe, only the actions of other humans, perhaps it is not surprising that few people are motivated to learn much math. This is important to consider when trying to improve the quality of mathematics education. The teaching of mathematics in schools may need to become more relevant to the lives of people, perhaps as a tool for understanding the actions of others and learning to make the best possible decisions in real life.

STUTTERING IN TONGUES

As mentioned earlier, mathematical abilities have become more or less synonymous with intelligence. Oratory feats have also been valued by many. People who are gifted with eloquence and fluency are likely to convince many more people than those without such gifts.

One of the most famous examples was the Greek orator Demosthenes, who was born in Athens in 384 BC. It may thus come as a surprise to most that Demosthenes suffered from severe stuttering. According to contemporary records, it was only through almost superhuman control that he was able to restrain it during his orations. But sometimes his speech would break down in severe stuttering, which was subsequently exploited by his enemies. In the year 322, Demosthenes committed suicide after he had fallen from grace, had lost his citizenship, and had been driven into exile.

Throughout most of our history, people with speech impediments such as stuttering have been ridiculed and seen as less able, significantly without any evidence of a link between stuttering and lower intelligence. Stuttering is a curious disorder that brain scientists are finally starting to understand, which may eventually lead to more effective treatments.

Throughout history many famous historic figures have suffered to a larger or lesser degree from stuttering: From Moses through the Roman emperor Claudius to the English king Charles I, as well as writers and freethinkers such as Lewis Carroll, Henry James, Winston Churchill, Charles Darwin, and Marilyn Monroe.

In 95% of sufferers, stuttering begins before the age of seven, where normal speech is interrupted by blocking, repeats, and prolongations of sounds. These interruptions are less recognizable than secondary effects that range from small minor hand movements to violent stamping and body spasms. At times it may seem as if the more the stutterer tries to speak, the less likely it is to happen.

Most stutterers live with a strong fear of stuttering and have developed a wide range of strategies to avoid it. Some pretend that they are mute and write their messages, while others substitute easy-to-pronounce words for difficult ones. For most stutterers, the affliction is an almost insurmountable handicap that interferes with normal communication.

Stuttering is found in approximately 1% of people, regardless of their native language. Thus, around two million Americans suffer from it, with four male stutterers to every female one. The clear male majority could indicate a strong genetic component. Studies in monozygotic twins have shown just over a 75% probability that both twins will have problems with stuttering if one does. In fraternal twins, the chance is a lot lower, just over a fourth, while the chance in ordinary siblings is below 25%.

Throughout recorded history stuttering has always existed. Even if around 80% of childhood stuttering disappears by itself around puberty, the remaining sufferers are left with such a serious handicap that therapies have been offered. Many of these are inefficacious and bizarre, to say the least. Demosthenes gave his own contribution to early anti-stuttering therapy with the interesting technique of reciting on the beach with pebbles in his mouth. He also forced himself to scale steep slopes with lead plates on his chest.

In the middle of the 1800s, some surgeons operated on stutterers' tongues, but without noticeable results. So-called modern explanations of stuttering have ranged from guilt, childhood traumas, sibling jealousy, hemispheric dominance, repressed anger, infantile sexual dispositions, deformations of tongue, lips, palate, jaw, or larynx, and chemical imbalances. These have led to therapies using medicine, hypnosis, biofeedback, electrical shock, healing, and psychoanalysis, none of which have helped much with the stuttering.

Brain Stuttering

Stuttering has thus remained enigmatic throughout most of human history. The last few decades have finally seen some scientific progress in understanding the underlying causes of stuttering. Human speech is a very complex process that involves around a hundred muscles. These muscles control the most important components for speech production: the larynx, which creates the sound; the pharynx, which creates the resonance; and the oral cavity, which modifies the sound. In addition, the effects of breathing also play an important role in creating sound.

Most people will talk at an average speech of 120 to 180 words per minute, which is the consequence of about 600 different configurations of those components. These configurations have to follow each other in a sequence. So it is quite a feat when children learn to talk, and perhaps even more surprising that so few children have trouble doing so.

Learning how and when to use the muscles involved in speech clearly depends on feedback from the ears. When we try to say something, we must be able to hear the sounds and do better next time. The auditive feedback comes through two routes: partly through a small delay via the air and partly through resonance from the skull and jaw. This is one of the reasons why our own voice sounds different to us when we listen to recordings of it.

In 1951, Bernard Lee published the observation that artificial stuttering can be induced by delaying the sound, using a tape recorder. This is similar to the experience of an echo in very long-distance telephone conversations that can make it almost impossible to have a normal conversation.

But stutterers have *fewer* problems when they hear this small delay. In addition, it was also found that their stuttering decreased when their own speech was masked by white noise of more than 85 decibels. It would also appear that slowing the speech helps them gain more control. This created a minor revolution in speech therapy that has helped many sufferers.

The idea is that it is possible to learn to control speech production and, through conscious strategies, change the movements of the muscles that create the difficult initial sounds. These sounds are stretched over time almost as with slow motion and are trained over and over again. When these sounds have been learned, they can be connected into syllables and words that are then combined into sentences.

So several pieces of evidence (including that most stutterers do *not* stutter when they whisper or sing) suggest that stuttering is caused by variations in the way the brain creates speech. This evidence has led to therapies that have helped some stutterers. But it is important to remember that many of the processes that underlie our ability to narrate our lives are not available for conscious introspection, and it can be difficult to see how we can control them. Furthermore, unan-swered questions remain about how speech and language in general are represented and generated in the brain.

Nevertheless, it is now clear that the notorious lack of eloquence shown by stutterers is not a reflection of their mental abilities. It is important that this knowledge and flexibility toward this serious handicap become integrated in our educational systems.

READING PROBLEMS

Reading disabilities and dyslexia can be as covert as stuttering is obvious. But their personal, economic, and social consequences are probably much more severe than those of stuttering in our society in which literacy is increasingly necessary. Dyslexia starts in childhood and remains a hard scientific problem. An understanding and effective therapy of the causes of dyslexia and reading disabilities could potentially have a huge influence on our society. Dyslexia exists in all age-groups, but most often develops when we learn to read as children, so we will focus on its possible causes in children.

Despite the fact that many young children get special help with learning to read, 5% to 15% of people across all cultures have severe problems with it. Like many other problems defined in terms of their symptoms, dyslexia's cause probably cannot be traced to just one fundamental deficit. On the contrary, dyslexia is probably an umbrella term for a group of underlying, connected problems that share the symptom of difficulty in learning to read.

Dyslexia is often defined as a specific deviation from the norm in terms of IQ score. But inability to read is not defined as *dyslexia* if the child's verbal and spatial IQ score is considerably lower than the average of 100. It *is* defined as dyslexia if reading problems are present and the spatial IQ score is much higher than the verbal IQ score, corresponding to more than two standard deviations. In children, IQ is meant to reflect the quotient between real and mental age. So it is said that a dyslexic child typically has a reading age that is one or two years less than children of the same age.

Although dyslexia often includes problems with spelling, it is primarily defined as *a measure of reading* (poor spellers are not necessarily dyslexic). Dyslexics read much more slowly than other people and, unlike normal readers, may even read words that are right side up and those that are upside down at the same slow speed.

Many researchers have seen the relationship among letters, words, and their pronunciation—phonological processing—as one of the most important hurdles in learning to read. Problems with this processing are seen as central in dyslexia. Many dyslexic children have major problems with rhyming and with dividing words into syllables. Dyslexics may also have memory problems; it has been said that they are able to hold fewer words in working memory than normal readers.

But of course reading also depends on our ability to visually decode words. Consider the large variation in fonts, including, for example, the difference between the type in this book and the handwritten words in a letter. In addition, consider the difference between words written only in CAPITALS and those written in a mixture of LoWErCASe and uPPeRcASE letTeRs. Despite the difference, we are quickly able to reduce these visual impressions to meaningful words. We are even aware of small changes in words that look similar, but have very different meanings, such as "read" and "reap."

A Brain Area for Visual Words?

Most of us are expert readers, but it is somewhat of an enigma that our brain can achieve expertise in such a recent invention. Given that the first alphabetic scripts were invented only a couple of thousand years ago, evolution has not had time to develop specialized brain parts for reading. Instead, reading is possibly the most important example of how the functions of brain regions can be redirected. In other words, reading is an example of how culture can shape the brain.

Over the last couple of years, brain scanning and neuropsychological experiments have demonstrated that reading takes over regions of the brain that would otherwise have other uses. This repudiates the previous claims of some researchers that the brain is capable of learning anything—that it is a blank sheet upon which anything can be written.

Quite on the contrary, we now know that the brain's learning possibilities are limited by our evolutionary history and the challenges that our common ancestors faced. Certain parts of the brain are specialized for the processing of one kind of sensory input, and not other kinds. In only very few cases can these areas be used for the processing of other sensory inputs. This means that flexibility of learning is often only possible in higher association areas and only to the extent that this new ability is related to the function of the existing region.

Reading is a complex skill that depends on many different brain areas spread over the whole brain. Words have to be recognized, and meaning has to be derived and integrated in longer sentences that allow us to pronounce the words and sentences. We are only slowly beginning to understand the details of how this process proceeds. We have gained understanding of the function of a region in the fusifom cortex on the underside of the brain between cortex and cerebellum. The region has been called the *visual word form area* and is a part of the visual regions that let us recognize objects.

The visual word form area appears to play a specific role in the early stages of reading in that it is only activated by visual words, and not, for example, by spoken words. In addition, this area seems to trigger the same amount of activity whether the person is reading real or pseudo words. Pseudo words are words such as "lyve" or "ryne" that follow the phonetic rules of English, so they are easy to pronounce, but are not found in the dictionary.

So it would appear that the visual word form area plays a more important role in decoding the visual form of a word rather than, for example, its meaning. People with lesions in this part of the brain are not able to read words at normal speed, but are sometimes able to decode the word, letter by letter. Paradoxically, these patients are sometimes fully capable of writing words, which they subsequently find very difficult to read again. They seldom have problems with hearing and understanding words, and are fully able to identify other visual objects such as faces or buildings.

Alphabetical Puns

Giving an adequate definition of "word" is surprisingly difficult. It is clear that a word has to contain letters from the alphabet used by the given language. As part of our mental development as children, we learn language and how to discern the words of the language. A bit later in development, we learn to read and write, and to decode and encode sounds from and to visual forms. Some ancient cultures, such as the Egyptians, chose to write with hieroglyphs in which, in its most simple form, every word corresponds to a visual shape, a hieroglyph. But having to learn all the visual shapes makes such a system impractical and time consuming. So new shapes were constructed as combinations of existing hieroglyphs. Eventually, the innovation of alphabetical script allowed a given language to be written from very few fundamental forms that can be combined to create the phonetic sound of a word.

How visual shapes become words depends on the culture. Japan has two writing systems: Kanji consists of symbols, and Kana consists of letters. Despite the difference in forms, some evidence suggests that the visual word region is present in the same part of the brain across cultures, although this remains controversial. This suggests that although we are not born with brain regions that specialize in reading, regardless of culture, we use the same brain regions when we learn to read.

The visual word form area becomes active whenever we see words, whether they are presented in the left or right part of the visual field. This area is equally active regardless of the words' case (lower- or uppercase letters) or font. So it has been suggested that the visual word form area represents the invariant visual form of a word.

The evidence comes from experiments using subliminal priming techniques in which words are presented for such brief intervals that participants are not conscious of having seen them. If a lowercase word such as "bear" is presented for around 33 milliseconds, followed by the same word in uppercase shown for significantly longer time, such as 300 milliseconds, the reaction time in a lexical-decision task is usually significantly reduced compared to that if an unrelated word (e.g., "loss") is used as a prime. This is called the *repetition priming effect.* Words such as "bear" and "BEAR" look very different because of the different shapes of some lower- and uppercase letters. Our capacity of perceiving the same word in any form can only be a result of learning. Neuroimaging experiments have found activity related to the repetition priming effect in the visual word form area, which suggests that this region could represent the invariant form of the word.

If this turns out to be true, it would be interesting to investigate what this region of the brain might do in those who have not yet learned to read, are learning to read, or have never learned to read. Although illiterates are unfortunately common in developing countries, it is difficult to find illiterates in the West who have never been exposed to words. Immigration laws conspire to make it difficult and expensive to study these groups with brain scanners.

Instead, a more feasible way to understand the development of reading is to study children who are learning to read. It has been shown that the visual word form area and nearby regions show an increase of activity as reading ability increases, so it has been named the *skill zone.*

Reading does not rely on activity solely in the visual word form area, but rather in a whole network of connected brain regions. Activity begins in the primary visual cortices and quickly spreads ventrally and dorsally to more anterior regions of the brain. This spreading wave of activity appears to code for increasingly abstract attributes of the visual input. A likely scenario is that of a serial decoding process in which lines of different orientation become letters that then become words that are recognized as real words, pseudo words, or non-words. But this process is only serial in the early stages and quickly becomes rather more complex with parallel processing of multiple spreading waves.

Using magnetoencephalography (MEG), we have recently been able to show that a part of the prefrontal cortex called the *inferior frontal gyrus* appears to be active before or at the same time as the visual word form area at around 130 milliseconds. This is a surprising finding given that the inferior frontal gyrus has previously been seen as part of the last steps of converting words to speech. Our results suggest that reading relies on top-down processing very early on when deciding whether a word can be pronounced or not.

This finding is related to how we learn words as infants. Our parents point and name an object, "cat," which creates an association between that object and a sound. We learn to decode the sounds that our parents make as speech and to discern the syllables and word units. In a sense, reading acts like a parasite on this system and is relying equally on both visual and auditory systems.

THUNDERSTONES VERSUS CHESS

The role of the visual form area in representing the invariant form of a word depends directly on the learning that typically occurs during childhood. This learning process can go awry in dyslexia, which ultimately manifests itself as a problem with fluent reading. This simple symptom can have many different underlying causes, which have become grouped under the convenient catch-all label of dyslexia. The causes of dyslexia are still unknown but one possible strategy might be to resolve the functional role of the visual word form area in dyslexia—and in evolutionary terms in general.

Although monkeys are generally thought to be unable to read, they are able to distinguish between different visual objects such as letters and words. Experiments using neurophysiological recordings of neural activity have shown that visual impressions are processed in different brain areas in relationship to a number of properties, such as their identity and their location in space. Similar to the object processing found in humans, dissociable brain regions in monkeys are related to the "what" and the "where" of visual objects. The ventral part of cortex in the fusiform cortex appears to be mostly concerned with the "what" of object processing, while more parietal regions appear to be concerned with the "where."

In humans, neuroimaging experiments have shown that words and faces are typically processed in cortical regions close to the regions that process visual impressions from the fovea of the retina. In contrast, it appears that buildings are processed in the cortical areas that are close to those areas that process visual impressions from the periphery of the retina. This may be related to the way we learn about them, with buildings mostly present in the periphery of vision and words and faces mostly present in the center of our vision.

Neurons in these brain regions appear to have different specializations. Some groups of neurons become active when parts of the face are shown, while other groups are most active when a face in profile is shown, and still others are active when the frontal face is shown. All three groups of neurons have been shown to connect to a further set of neurons that become active to the invariant properties of a face. This observation means that the activity is not dependent on factors such as the portion, size, or viewing position of the object. So it has been proposed that a hierarchy of neurons exists in which the processing becomes ever more abstract, such that neurons at the top of the hierarchy represent the identity of an object.

The thunderstones described in the beginning of the chapter are examples of visual shapes that we can learn to recognize. It takes time to become expert in recognizing thunderstones because they can be found in many different shapes. Their archetypal shape is an oblong, pointed-on-one-end cylinder with a diameter of about half a centimeter and a typical length of 8 to 9 centimeters. The ravages of time have broken and changed the shape of many thunderstones, but the color is a good indicator, because they are golden when wet.

With the necessary motivation and desire, I became expert at spotting thunderstones, which then seemed to almost jump out from the other pebbles. Given enough time and training, most people are able to become experts at quickly distinguishing between similar visual objects. But finding thunderstones is an example of a complicated task that we have yet to develop good computer algorithms to solve except in very simple cases. It is remarkable that this is more difficult for computers than playing chess.

LIMITS FOR LEARNING

Learning to spot thunderstones shares many properties with learning to read. It is likely that one or more areas of my brain will respond maximally when I see a thunderstone and not when I see words. These areas may well represent the invariant form of thunderstones, so they are a direct function of learning. Both words and thunderstones are processed in those brain areas that have access to the central part of our visual impressions. Both types of objects depend on already existing brain areas whose spatial placement and extent may be partly determined by genetic influences. So, for example, the visual word form area is invariably close to areas that are concerned with early visual processing and would not be expected to be found in the frontal parts of the brain. This is why we are limited in what we can learn and in the possible variations of behavior. We are unable to learn to see infrared light because our sensory receptors and brain have not been shaped by evolution to sense infrared light.

This also means that we can now explain why children always go through a phase in which they write letters such as w and m upside down and mirrored, and why they find it difficult to distinguish between the lowercase letters p, q, b, and d. These letters are mirrored and rotated variations of each other. Our visual system is very good at reducing this variance and to recognize the letter as variations of just one invariant form. But this is not helpful in reading, so children have to learn to explicitly fight this tendency and learn to see the letters as different shapes.

So reading is a good example of cultural learning that we can hope to improve with a better understanding of the underlying brain processes. But better learning strategies will need a better understanding of the pleasures, desires, and emotions that are crucial to ensure the necessary motivation for learning.

PLAYFUL RATS

Like other animals, humans use play as the natural way to learn. We know remarkably little about which parts of the brain are specifically involved in play. Thus, we do not know for sure why adults play less than children do. It is difficult to design experiments that can identify active brain regions during play. It is also difficult to identify well-defined tasks that include elements that resemble the unspoiled play we experienced as children, in which we lose the sense of time and place.

Such a state might be called *fluid absorption* to reflect the kind of dissolution of self that is present in activities that afford us fundamental pleasure with no promise of external reward. One could compare this experience with skiing or snowboarding, but it is also in many ways an intense feeling not unlike satisfying sex. It is not obvious how to measure this state of fluid absorption in a brain scanner. To do so would require that the participants perform tasks that are similar to those that evoke fluid absorption, but without actually experiencing the dynamic process.

Of course, one might examine other species. For example, rats and mice are fundamentally different in their styles of play. Rats are keen to engage in playing and play-fighting, while mice spend very little time, if any, engaged in such activities. This could be why it is much easier to teach rats tricks, and why many complex scientific experiments rely on rats rather than mice. The brains of rats and mice are very similar, but there obviously are small but significant genetic differences that make rats' brains much more adept at playing and probably also at learning.

Play expands the behavioral repertoire of humans as well as other animals. By imitating and simulating other beings, we learn new ways to do things that provide joy in the doing. Dance, drama, and sports include these elements of fluid absorption. People instinctively find these activities pleasurable to do and to observe, even when they are not experts at them.

How can we learn to use this element of playfulness in learning processes? Good learning must stem from internal motivation or desires, because otherwise it is difficult to see why anyone would voluntarily spend a long time mastering a complex task. It is vital to support children in learning to control this internal motivation. Parents should not be unduly worried if their children spend time with computers and computer games. That which constitutes a good computer game is exactly the element of fluid absorption, which creates the sustained motivation to attempt to continue playing to prolong the experience.

Rather than providing a specific reward, play appears to constitute its own reward. A classic study investigated reward processing in children. Two groups of nursery-school children were handed a set of crayons and some paper, and were asked to draw to their hearts' content. One group was told that they would receive a handsome certificate for their drawings, while the other group was promised nothing. In due course, the crayons and paper were put away for two weeks. When they were restored, the children who had received a certificate now displayed a radically reduced enthusiasm for drawing, particularly in comparison with the other group of children, who were as enthusiastic as before. Many other studies have shown that when we are rewarded for activities we do for pleasure, we tend to lose interest in them.

A key element of learning to control internal reward is learning to focus the search for this experience and to incorporate variety in the process. It is not adaptive to focus all one's energy on mastering computer games or sports when successful social interactions require other important skills such as reading, eloquence, and even mathematics. The arts of good parenting and teaching include providing elements of fluid absorption to learning situations.

We still do not know much about which brain areas partake in the experiences of play and fluid absorption. One obvious possibility is that they might involve the very same areas that are important for other pleasures and desires. The brain clearly produces internal rewards that can be triggered by other systems involving taste, smell, sex, and drugs.

Although not many would spend as much time as I did to become an expert thunderstone collector, I like to think that it was time well spent. I got to spend time with my grandfather, and came to understand early that, given the right motivation, we can learn almost any task. Effective learning is foremost about having the necessary motivation to find and internalize knowledge in the best possible way. This can take the form of explicit teaching, but can also occur without it.

● ● ● HAPPINESS LESSONS

"Practice makes perfect" has a firm basis in cognitive neuroscience. Frequent repetition solidifies skills of all sorts.

Beware of assuming that gender differences are inherent; they are often purely societal in origin.

Play is a crucial component in children's learning—and for adults, too! Fluid absorption is a state of happiness.

FURTHER READING

In a very deep sense, learning is lifelong, but certain things come easier if they are started early. Vision and other sensory learning are clearly some of the most important abilities that can subsequently be built upon. Stuttering is an example of what can easily go wrong, and a good guide is the following book: Bobrick, B. (1995). *Knotted Tongues. Stuttering in History and the Quest for a Cure.* New York, NY: Simon & Schuster.

Mathematics is also a somewhat sore problem for many. For intriguing information regarding this important skill, I highly recommend the following book: Dehaene, S. (1997). *The Number Sense. How the Mind Creates Mathematics.* Oxford: Oxford University Press.

All of this learning would not be able to occur without pleasure, desire, and emotion, but it is important to be cautious of oversimplified ideas about rewards and punishment in learning. The following book is an interesting part of this cautionary tale: Lepper, M. R. & Greene, D. (1978). *The Hidden Costs of Reward.* Morristown, NJ: Lawrence Erlbaum.

8

MADNESS

Malignant Desires

To see a World in a Grain of Sand
And a Heaven in a Wild Flower,
Hold Infinity in the palm of your hand
And Eternity in an hour.

William Blake (1757–1827)

In November 2005, the Dalai Lama was invited to speak at the annual meeting of the Society for Neuroscience in Washington, D.C. Although this event was not without controversy, he surprised many scientists with his remarkable open-mindedness, particularly concerning the validity of neuroscientific enquiry. The Dalai Lama spoke of how humans have "much conflicting emotion, much bad emotion, jealousy, anger, fear. This is our great troublemaker." He confessed that he "still feels anger and fear." He said that meditation can help, but that he was not averse to other paths. He volunteered himself as a patient if neuroscientists wanted to pursue easier ways to quell the "troublemakers of the mind."

The pursuit of happiness is a preoccupation for many people and probably has been since the dawn of mankind. Yet few of us come close to achieving this state with any regularity. And even when happiness finally descends upon us, we often only realize it after the fact.

MALIGNANT SADNESS

Depression is a very common disorder, which can affect other internal organs including the heart. It is often closely related to excessive hypochondria, although that is not the *cause* of depression. Depression is deadly to a degree that results in suicide for approximately one out of ten clinically depressed people. Although, about a third of us will go through a major depression, most people do not like to talk about depression. Depression and other mental illnesses remain very much taboo, unlike physical illnesses such as flu and tonsillitis.

This taboo is linked historically with a couple of factors that have caused many people to try to hide and deny a clinical depression rather than seek treatment. One is that Western medicine traditionally has seen the body as separate from the mind, which means that illnesses of the mind have been treated differently than have the illnesses of the body. But even if it may still be difficult to accept, scientific evidence clearly shows that our mental activity, be it normal or abnormal, is a product of biological activity in the brain.

Also, the overwhelming complexity of the brain has previously interfered with diagnosing and treating mental illness. Historically, the mentally ill have been sent to mental hospitals where they were often treated worse than criminals.

The English biologist Lewis Wolpert did not try to hide his own depression, but instead used it as the basis for a fine small book on the topic. Wolpert frankly recounts how he was unable to think about anything but suicide during his depression. His most pressing initial problem was that he did not have a painfree and certain way to kill himself. He gathered a large supply of sleeping pills and heart medicine, but worried that he would awaken to find himself even worse. He contemplated smashing his locked hospital window and jumping from the seventh floor, but knew that his fear of heights would make this impossible. While at home during the day, he kept fantasizing about running his head through the glass window to cut his throat.

When Wolpert's wife found out about these suicidal thoughts, she became furious, and asked him to consider the unbearable situation he would create for their children and her. In return, she promised to help him commit suicide if his condition had not improved within a year. Luckily, he trusted her and slowly started the recovery that almost invariably will occur after some time, and which for most people rarely lasts more than a year.

Pills or Psychotherapy?

There is hope for relief from depression. As we have increased our understanding of the functions of the brain, we also have become better equipped to treat mental illness. New antidepressants such as the so-called serotonin-uptake blockers, including Prozac and Cipralex, are examples of treatment. Although it would be wonderful if these pills alone could cure depression, some researchers doubt that it is possible.

The brain is so complex that it is unlikely that a single pill will be able to restore its balance. The more likely solution lies in investigating and restoring the imbalances that the depression is a symptom of. It is also important to distinguish between the symptoms and the underlying biological and psychological causes. Correctly diagnosing mental illness is difficult, so it is not surprising that the precise biological and psychological causes can be even harder to unravel.

However, this difficulty does not preclude the existence of countless explanatory models and theories for depression. Many doctors have a natural predilection for biological explanations for depression, which may be true when pushed to extremes. But because we do not yet fully understand how the mind emerges from biological and psychological constraints such as brain activity, these explanations do not help enough.

Although the brain is created from our genes, they do not contain enough code for all connections in the brain and for environmental conditions. Influences in the uterus and early childhood, known as *psychological* factors, must also play a significant role. They are likely to be as important as neurobiological factors, so any explanation and treatment method must take them into consideration. The diversity of factors that contribute to depression means that different kinds of treatments have their respective strengths and weaknesses.

But we do not yet have scientific evidence for the superiority of one method over all others.

Specifically, scientific evidence does not support the contention that pills are better than psychotherapy—or vice versa. Some researchers even doubt that antidepressants are significantly better than placebos, especially if the often-serious side effects of antidepressants are considered. A meta-analysis of clinical studies of depression has shown that the very small difference between the effectiveness of placebos and antidepressants may be interpreted such that more than half the effect of antidepressants can be ascribed to placebo effects while only around a quarter of the effect can be ascribed to the active ingredients. This interpretation is, of course, contested by the pharmaceutical industry.

Nevertheless, emerging literature questions the efficacy and safety of some antidepressants. One example is an article in the *British Medical Journal* that questions whether the scientific evidence supports using certain antidepressants in children and adolescents. The article showed worrisome problems in how clinical studies of depression are carried out and reported. The article also showed that, by most criteria, placebo treatments are at least as effective as antidepressants. The authors conclude that, given the serious side effects of antidepressants, the scientific evidence does not support using antidepressants in children and adolescents.

Other studies have shown that the possibility of increased mortality as a consequence of antidepressants should not be rejected. In other words, it is not possible to reject that antidepressants can contribute to the suicides of depressed children and adolescents. This has led the U.S. Food and Drug Administration to ask for a strong warning to be included with antidepressants.

Time is perhaps the most important factor for depression. Probably about 80% of all depressed patients—even without treatment—will come to feel as well as before they became depressed. However, recovery can take up to a year or longer.

Evidence suggests that the best treatment for depression is a combination of time, pills, and psychotherapy. There is also the possibility of treatment through direct action on the brain; an experimental treatment along these lines is detailed here.

THE DEPRESSIVE BRAIN

Quite a few studies have now carried out brain scanning of depressed patients, on and off medication before, during, and after clinical depression. The results show a complex network of brain regions involved in emotion and hedonic experience, which seems to account for the fact that such a complicated illness as depression should have a multitude of underlying factors. Given that depression is primarily diagnosed on the basis of symptoms, it is likely that depression is common to a series of different brain states that just happen to evoke the same symptoms.

One common symptom in depression and other mental illnesses is *anhedonia,* the pronounced lack of pleasure. Depressed patients rarely find much pleasure in anything, including things they normally would, such as family, food, or sex. The anhedonia seen in depressed patients is a good example of the importance of pleasure to our everyday well-being.

Among the many brain regions found in neuroimaging studies, depression shows up most in a region called the *subgenual cingulate cortex*, which is intimately connected to the orbitofrontal cortex. This brain region has also been shown to be an important part of the brain's resting network, which is active even at rest. Studies in monkeys have shown that neurons in this brain region change their activity when the monkey is about to fall asleep. In addition, as shown in earlier chapters, activity in the medial orbitofrontal cortex is related to the monitoring of the pleasantness and unpleasantness of stimuli. So dysregulation of the activity in these regions would seem likely to affect the subjective hedonic experience and perhaps even lead to anhedonia.

Based on these findings, the American neuroscientist Helen Mayberg used deep brain stimulation in the subgenual cingulate cortex for patients with treatment-resistant depression. Initially, the treatment resulted in sustained remission of depression in four of six patients. Given the strong placebo component in depression, it is too early to say to what extent this might help others.

But the problem is not only the lack of pleasure but also malignant desire. In the same way as the principle of selective satiation makes sure that we get enough food variety, a related mechanism is called *incentive motivation*. For example, it makes sure that if we find peanuts and chocolate equally rewarding, we are more likely to stick with the one we started on than to change. It is popularly known as the salted-peanuts phenomenon, because most people know what it is like to be unable to stop eating peanuts until the bowl is empty. Presumably, the mechanism has been selected by evolution so we will not expend much energy constantly changing our behavior. Depression and other forms of mental illness might involve an abnormal variation of this mechanism whereby one's thoughts keep focusing on the same negative thoughts rather than changing to positive ones.

The coming years should tell us more about the many ways in which the depressed brain might be different from the normal brain. Because the normal brain falls into depressive patterns sooner rather than later, many of these changes have to be rather subtle. It is clear that there is a genetic component to depression. More thorough and well-controlled studies might be able to use these genetic differences to uncover interesting new findings with regard to both brain anatomy and brain activity.

THE VERGE OF INSANITY

The flipside of depression is the mania that characterizes bipolar patients, who alternate between depression and mania. Bipolar disorder and other types of madness are likely to form part of the fundamental human condition. These days, modern medicine tries to diagnose and treat those humans whose behavior is potentially dangerous to themselves and others. The diagnosis of advanced madness relies on symptoms, such as when patients insist they hear imaginary voices or are followed by imaginary people. Instead of "madness," we now use more clinical names such as schizophrenia and paranoia to cover what is claimed to be more precise symptoms.

Throughout history, many famous artists are among the people who have suffered from bipolar disorder, such as the writer Virginia Woolf, the poet John Keats, and the composer Robert Schumann. A hallmark of these artists is the variability in the quality of their creations, with many of their indisputable masterpieces appearing to coincide with their manic periods. This has led some researchers to propose a close link between madness and creativity, and that this link can be found in the variations of personality types. The American psychologist Branden Thornhill-Miller has shown how this link is part of a triad of personality traits, which also includes proneness to deep religious experiences.

Some people who suffer from bipolar disorder and schizophrenia will sometimes experience what appear to be deep, sudden insights into the structure of the universe. In addition, patients with temporal epilepsy will sometimes attribute cosmic meaning to events that occurred during an epileptic attack. Of course the link between the propensity for deep religious insights and certain brain disorders does not show that religiosity exists only as a function of brain activity in some brain region such as the temporal lobes. Rather, this finding clearly shows that mechanisms for those religious experiences are common across all human cultures.

Madness and normality often are not far apart. An excellent example is the story of two researchers who contributed to the first edition of *The Oxford English Dictionary* (which took more than 70 years and a large number of volunteers to finish).

The Great Dictionary

Lexicography is the noble art of defining words, and it requires a certain noble temperament to dedicate years of one's life to finding the roots of words. That is especially true if one insists that a dictionary is not only a list of different meanings of a word, but more akin to a biography that allows the reader to trace a word from its conception in literature and read examples of its many uses. When the learned English Philological Society decided in 1857 to compile a dictionary, the only way that this gargantuan task could be realized was by sharing the task among many different correspondents spread around the globe. This supposedly would allow for a quicker and more efficient trawling of the extensive literature.

James Murray was born into a poor family in the village of Denholm near Hawick in the Scottish Borders. His poor circumstances forced him to leave school at the age of 14. But this did not stop him from amassing an extraordinary amount of knowledge with a determination that would eventually lead him to Oxford. When he was 32 years old, Murray was admitted to the Philological Society. In the end, his obvious talents and connections led to what became his mission in life: the creation of the great English dictionary. He steered the large dictionary project for over 36 years. The story goes that for more than 20 of those years, Murray had invited Dr. W.C. Minor, one of the most productive correspondents, to Oxford to discuss finer aspects of lexicography. Minor had always declined, even though he lived in Berkshire, only an hour away from Oxford by train.

Finally, Murray decided to take matters into his own hands by taking the train to Berkshire. At the station, he was picked up by a cab horse that brought him through country roads to a large red brick mansion at the end of a poplar-covered avenue. A butler led Murray to a sizable library where a small man sat almost hidden behind a rather large mahogany desk. Murray introduced himself and added—almost like Stanley in search of the source of the Nile—"and you must be Dr. Minor, I presume."

After a long, awkward pause, the small man cleared his throat and paused to fiddle with his glasses before he said: "I am sorry to inform you, Sir, that I am not Dr. Minor. I am the superintendent here at the Broadmoor Asylum for the Criminally Insane. Dr. Minor is of course here but he is a patient of this asylum and has been so for 25 years. He is our longest staying resident."

Roots of Madness

William Chester Minor was born in 1834 to American missionaries in Sri Lanka (then known as Ceylon). When he was three, his mother died from lung tuberculosis and his father remarried. At 14, William was sent to America to study at the Yale University, where he stayed for 15 years, until he was fully trained as a surgeon.

Minor was obsessed by what he later called his *animal instincts*. By age 29, sex and guilt had already started to torture Minor in a way that is sometimes seen in the very devout. This perhaps contributed to the fateful incident that was to shape his life.

In the same year, 1863, Minor felt patriotic enough about his adopted country to enlist in the Civil War, which was in full force. At his request, he served as a surgeon in the hard-fought battle in Orange County in Virginia. Even normal humans can be struck by madness when they are faced with the horrors of war. It is all too easy to imagine how these horrific events may have marked Minor.

In any case, Minor's character changed in the years following the war, and he started to frequent houses of ill repute. He also so devoted himself to compulsive thoughts that he eventually got committed to a mental hospital and was forced to retire from the army. Then, in 1871, Minor decided to go to Europe to start a new life.

Murder on Lambeth Marsh

Minor did not get the fresh start in England that he hoped for. Instead he continued to give free rein to his baser instincts with prostitutes and found it hard to control his ever-more-pressing obsessive thoughts. He started carrying a gun for fear of Irish men who, he was convinced, followed him and forced him to unmentionable acts each night.

Early on a February morning in 1872, Minor shot and killed a poor brewer. The police quickly arrested Minor, who confessed immediately. In the trial, Minor was judged to be insane when he committed the crime and was condemned to confinement in a mental hospital.

The American Embassy arranged to have books brought to Minor's cell. Tormented by guilt, Minor gave a large sum of money to the widow of his victim. The madness remained, especially at night, but leveled off as time passed. Volunteering to the great English dictionary project also seemed to have a calming effect. However, this did not prevent him, late in life, from cutting off his penis. This presumably was linked to what may have been going on with his victim's widow, whom he paid to bring him books from London on a regular basis. Minor's surgical workmanship made sure he survived the amputation. When his sentence expired, he returned to the United States, where he died in 1920, 5 years after Murray.

Photos show that Minor and Murray looked remarkably alike with their long white beards. They shared a deep love for words, which especially for schizophrenics come to rule their lives. Although Minor was excessively mad and religious, he managed to leave a lasting contribution to one of the towering achievements of lexicography.

Almost every day, I cycle past Murray's old house in Oxford on Banbury Road 78, which contained the *Scriptorium,* where Murray ran the dictionary project. I wonder what separated this self-taught Scottish polymath from the mad American surgeon. Minor's madness would probably have been classified as schizophrenia today, but is this too convenient a label? In the world of words, Minor found the freedom to escape the tribulations of madness. The Oxford English Dictionary project may have given Murray honor and glory, but it also became a self-elected prison for life, which was not altogether different from Minor's cell.

Madness of the Prophet

Schizophrenia is diagnosed on the basis of a long list of symptoms that include hearing voices in one's head. The illness most often manifests itself in patients during their early twenties. Schizophrenic patients often are so disabled that they are unable to function in normal social contexts. In earlier times, this state was often just called *madness.*

At first sight, madness appears to be pouring out of the works of the English painter and poet William Blake. This apparent madness takes the form of demons, monsters, and other strange night creatures seemingly cut from the very material of nightmares. Other contemporary artists tried to portray London, but only Blake's swirling wood engravings truly captured the energy of those days. This energy was a constant companion from his early years, when apparitions of angels and inner visions made him devote his life to art. Reality appears to have lost its appeal for Blake early on. Instead he spent more and more of his time in the world of imagination.

From the first illuminated poetry collections *Songs of Innocence* from 1789 and *Songs of Experience* from 1794 to the prophetical books from the 1780s and 1790s to the late, unfinished illustrations of Dante, Blake managed to create a very personal and original universe, but to awful reviews. For example, in 1809 one reviewer wrote that Blake was an "unfortunate lunatic, whose personal inoffensiveness secures him from confinement." Blake's contemporaries were so appalled by the insanity of his work that few found anything of lasting value in his distinctive blend of drawings, text, colors, and poems. It was only more than a century later, with the large postwar generations' experimentation with drugs and their influence on the "doors of perception," that a larger audience came to appreciate Blake's work. Since then, he has been celebrated as a visionary and deeply original artist who continues to inspire other artists.

Madness can take many forms, but these days modern medicine tries to diagnose and treat those whose behavior is a potential danger to themselves and others. This diagnosis is seldom called *madness* these days, but by rather clinical names such as schizophrenia, which presumably is a better description of the symptoms.

Under these clinical criteria, no doubt Blake would have been offered various drugs and psychotherapy, which help relieve the everyday worries of people who otherwise would be incapable of enjoying life. But our world would have been a lesser place with a Blake on psychopharmacological drugs. Instead we have Blake's celebration of antirationality, as in the masterly portrait of Newton lost in thought over his geometric figures. There is method to Blake's madness, and depths and extremes in his writings and art that very few will come to experience outside art.

INSANE BRAINS

For many years, researchers have tried to find out whether schizophrenic and normal brains differ anatomically. Although the scientific literature is full of examples of statistically significant differences, very few of these findings have endured. One is that many schizophrenics smoke a lot, perhaps because nicotine helps them to self-medicate, so it appears likely that the nicotinic receptors in the brain play an important role.

Brain researchers thought that one of the more certain findings was from the Danish neuroscientist Bente Pakkenberg. By investigating the brains of normal and schizophrenic humans post-mortem, she found a reduction of neurons in the mediodorsal part of the thalamus, which is a part of the brain with connections to the prefrontal cortex. The finding would seem to be meaningful because many of the symptoms of schizophrenia may be explained in terms of abnormal activity in the prefrontal cortex. But counting cells is not an exact science, and some recent doubts have colored the significance of this finding. When the Scottish psychiatrist Tom Cullen carried out the largest postmortem study of schizophrenic and normal brains, he failed to replicate the earlier finding of a significant difference between the two groups. Other research groups since then have also failed to replicate the results.

Similar to depression, schizophrenia is probably not just one illness, but rather a name given to symptoms arising variously from changes in activity in many different brain regions. So perhaps it is not surprising that brain imaging of schizophrenic brains has found differences compared to normal brains, but it is difficult to know to what degree these differences reflect activity related to schizophrenia. It may also just be that the findings reflect small differences between groups with rather diffuse symptoms. For example, one finding is that schizophrenic patients apparently have problems predicting even simple motor movements, although it is highly unlikely that this deficit alone would explain schizophrenia. Another observation is the anhedonia and changed experience of reward that is seen in almost all forms of mental illness.

Depression, mania, schizophrenia, and other mental illnesses have caused so much suffering to so many people that we need all the help we can get. Even if there is darkness in the depth of the malignant emotions, and suicide seems like the only way out, it is important to get correct and timely information about how to recover. There is always hope—even if it may at times seem like only a glimmer. At the end of the day, it is other people who make it worth staying on and who can help us back to the pleasure and happiness of life.

But what is the relationship between desire, pleasure, and happiness? Might happiness be best described as pleasure without desire, a state of contentment and indifference? Such a state is perhaps akin to the kind of bliss that Buddhists seek through meditation. If so, it is possible that neuroscientists may one day find ways to help induce this state. Then we might have a chance of a true utilitarian society in which overall happiness can be maximized, as the eighteenth century philosopher Jeremy Bentham proposed. The question of whether such a society would be desirable and even pleasurable remains to be answered.

● ● ● HAPPINESS LESSONS

Don't give up hope. Most obstacles are usually not as permanent as they initially seem to be. You may feel like things will never change and that you're doomed, but that perception is as much or more of a mood than an unyielding reality. Negative thoughts are just thoughts, not reality.

As neuroscience and psychology advance further, year by year, more helpful options become available for those suffering mental problems.

The lack of pleasure in mental illness

Mental illnesses such as depression and eating disorders afflict many people and are characterized by the lack of pleasure, anhedonia. This would suggest that the reward systems of the brain have become unbalanced. Investigating the many faces of pleasure can therefore help understand when and why pleasure disappears.

The pleasures of the brain consist of many conscious and nonconscious processes such as liking, wanting, and learning. Through the systematic scientific study of the relationship between these subcomponents, we can hopefully learn to rebalance the brain.

Take as an example addiction, which has been proposed to be characterized by how brain processes involved in wanting take over from those involved in liking. An extreme example is how a rat will continue to self-stimulate at all costs, even at the expense of eating, drinking, or sleeping, and apparently without any "liking."

In many cases, the unbalanced brain may rebalance itself with time but often this may require active intervention. Some of the more radical interventions can be through brain stimulation or pills but behavioral therapies can also be remarkably effective to rebalance the brain

FURTHER READING

Mental illness is a part of life for many, more than most would think. An excellent short introduction to depression is this book: Wolpert, L. (2000). *Malignant Sadness: The Anatomy of Depression*. London: Free Press. Interesting insights in bipolar disorder seen from the inside can be found in Jamison, K. R. (1995). *An Unquiet Mind. A Memoir of Moods and Madness.* New York, NY: Alfred A. Knopf.

The Oxford English Dictionary is described in more detail in this very readable book: Winchester, S. (1999). *The Surgeon of Crowthorne: A Tale of Murder, Madness and the Oxford English Dictionary.* Oxford: Oxford University Press.

9

STIMULANTS

Pain and Pleasure, Food and Drugs

Description of man: dependence, desire for independence, need.

Blaise Pascal (1623–1662)

This chapter considers those plant-based stimulants that people have used to help them through their humdrum existence. Tea, coffee, tobacco, and alcohol are just some of the many stimulants that are desired and consumed daily around the globe, even though most of us know that excessive use easily leads to abuse and addiction. The brain is central in this abuse and addiction, and we now know that the brain activity that corresponds to stimulants is remarkably similar to that which corresponds to food and sex.

In this chapter, we also investigate how other cultures use stimulants that our culture classifies as illegal. In this context, it is worth noting that the current state of affairs came about mostly through accidents of history—so it might be worth rethinking the status quo. But let us start with pleasure.

PLEASURE AND HOMEOSTASIS IN THE BRAIN

The essential energy to sustain life, as well as many pleasures of life, come from food intake. Although the necessary homeostatic regulation and consummatory behavior required to maintain it is hard-wired in even brainless species, it is much harder for mammals to regulate our feeding, because we must maintain a stable body temperature in a wide variety of hostile climates, which in turn requires intricate neural circuits.

The relative sophistication of foraging in higher primates compared to other mammals indicates that significant parts of our large brains are dedicated to the required motivational, emotional, and cognitive processing, and that mental processes related to food intake may indeed underlie other higher functions. The special importance of food in human life is underlined by the predominance of food symbols and metaphors in human expressions across cultures, as described by French anthropologist Claude Lévi-Strauss. Similarly, elaborate social constructions concerning purity and taboo of foods exist across all human cultures, as the English anthropologist Mary Douglas described in detail.

Of course, food intake and choice are a fundamental and frequent part of human life. The American biologist Jared Diamond has convincingly shown how food has played a major part in the cultural evolution of nonfood systems such as ritual, religion, and social exchange, as well as in the advancement of technology, the development of cities, illnesses, warfare, agriculture, and domestication.

The brain controls our food intake by obtaining sensory information about a food, evaluating its desirability, and choosing the appropriate behavior. Part of this process is closely linked to simple homeostatic regulation, in common with that of other animals, as was demonstrated in numerous experiments with rats. Fundamentally, such regulation depends on activity in the brainstem, and on molecular processes. However, food intake in humans is not regulated by homeostatic processes alone, as is illustrated by our easy overindulgence in sweet foods beyond our homeostatic needs, and by rising obesity levels (nearly 20% of the U.S. population is classified as clinically obese).

This tendency to overindulge is because food intake is determined by the interaction between homeostatic regulation and hedonic processes, that is, the pleasure derived from consumption. This complex sub-cortical and cortical processing involves higher-order processes such as learning, memory, planning, and expectation. It also gives rise to the conscious experience of the sensory properties of the food (such as its identity, intensity, temperature, fat content, and viscosity), as well as to the valence elicited by the food (including, most importantly, the hedonic experience it gives).

Evidence from recent neuroimaging studies links regions of the human brain (in particular, the orbitofrontal cortex) to various aspects of food intake, and especially to the representation of the subjective experience of pleasantness. These findings appear for the first time to give us a solid basis for the further exploration of the brain systems involved in the conscious experience of pleasure and reward, and provide a unique method for studying the hedonic quality of human experience.

This hedonic experience is related to *qualia,* "the hard problem of consciousness," which some philosophers believe will never be amenable to scientific analysis. And yet, as demonstrated below, recent neuroimaging of the mechanisms behind food intake suggests that this line of scientific inquiry may eventually yield important insights into the core of subjective experience.

Chocolate Milk and Tomato Juice

Food intake is such a common act that most people rarely think about the complexities it involves. Yet it is a precisely controlled act that can be potentially fatal if the wrong decision is taken—for instance, to swallow toxins, microorganisms, or nonfood objects on the basis of erroneously determining the sensory properties of the food. Human beings have therefore developed elaborate food behaviors aimed at balancing conservative and life-preserving strategies with occasional novelty seeking in the hope of discovering new sources of nutrients.

Food intake is thus a highly complicated process dependent on many contributing factors in which learning plays a very important role. Essentially, the process must provide the right balance of carbohydrates, fats, amino acids, vitamins, and minerals (apart from sodium) to sustain life.

When we have eaten, hours pass before the food is broken down into those nutrients that give us enough energy to go on. As a result, if we consider the question of controlling food intake, we have to take into account the significant delays before the effects of consumption are manifest, caused by the relatively slow metabolic processes. This means that the regulatory neural systems controlling food intake must include sophisticated mechanisms so that we can predict when a meal should be started and finished.

Everyone is familiar with the important mechanisms for "selective satiety." We have all experienced the feeling of having plenty of room and desire for the dessert despite being completely full from the main course. From an evolutionary perspective, this has the clear advantage of allowing us and other animals to obtain a sufficiently wide variety of nutrients.

Selective satiety (or "sensory-specific satiety," as it is also known) is a particularly useful phenomenon for studying affective representation in the brain, because it provides a way of altering the affective value of a stimulus without modifying its physical attributes. As a result, any differences observed between the representation of a particular food stimulus in the brain before and after satiety can be attributed to the change in the impact of the reward, or the reward value. This is a control for possible confounds, such as increases in thirst, gastric distension, and changes in blood glucose levels after feeding, because the neural responses are measured to both foods, that is also to food not eaten in the meal. Selective satiety effects are strongest when using quite different foods such as tomato juice (savory) and chocolate milk (sweet).

Our research group used functional magnetic resonance imaging to investigate the neural mechanisms related to selective satiety. This process allowed us to identify the neural correlates of subjective pleasantness. As always, however, the devil is in the details, and a more precise description of the experiment follows (Figure 9.1).

To motivate the participants properly, we asked them to refrain from eating for at least 6 hours before the experiment. They were prescreened to ensure that they found both tomato juice and chocolate milk pleasant. We also ensured that they were not overweight, dieting, or even planning to go on a diet. Both chocolate milk and tomato juice were chosen to be palatable at room temperature. The clear difference in their flavor and texture helps to facilitate selective satiety effects and minimizes the likelihood of the participants' developing a generalized satiety to both of the liquid foods.

For the first part of the experiment, the participants were placed in the brain imaging scanner and scanned while being presented with the two liquid foods as well as a tasteless control solution, each delivered to the participant's mouth through three tubes held between the lips. The tasteless control solution consisted of water added to the main ionic components of saliva. In other words, rather than using water, which is known to be rewarding to hungry participants, we used artificial saliva as a control—a fact that was not divulged to the participants, as this might have altered their experience of an otherwise rather neutral solution.

The trick of neuroimaging is to present the various stimuli repeatedly until statistically significant brain responses are obtained. Our experiment used a block design where

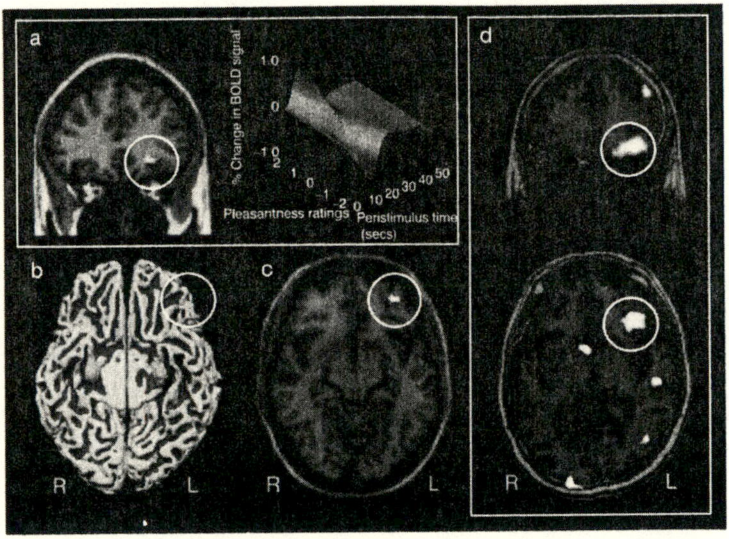

Figure 9.1 Hedonic experience in the brain. (a) A neuroimaging study using selective satiation found that mid-anterior parts of the orbitofrontal cortex are correlated with the subjects' subjective pleasantness ratings of the foods throughout the experiment. (b) Additional evidence for the role of the orbitofrontal cortex in subjective experience comes from another neuroimaging experiment investigating the supra-additive effects of combining the umami tastants. The figure shows the region of mid-anterior orbitofrontal cortex showing synergistic effects (rendered on the ventral surface of human cortical areas with the cerebellum removed). The perceived synergy is unlikely to be expressed in the taste receptors themselves and the activity in the orbitofrontal cortex may thus reflect the subjective enhancement of umami taste which must be closely linked to subjective experience. (c) Adding strawberry odor to a sucrose taste solution makes the combination significantly more pleasant than the sum of each of the individual components. The supra-linear effects reflecting the subjective enhancement were found to significantly correlate with the activity in a lateral region of the left anterior orbitofrontal cortex, which is remarkably similar to that found in the other experiments. (d) These findings were strengthened by findings using deep brain stimulation (DBS) and magnetoencephalography (MEG). Pleasurable subjective pain relief for chronic pain in a phantom limb in a patient was causally induced by effective deep brain stimulation in the brainstem. When using MEG to directly measure the concomitant changes in the rest of the brain, a significant change in power was found in the mid-anterior orbitofrontal cortex.

each block lasted 16 seconds. At the beginning of each block, a tiny amount (0.75 ml) of either the liquid foods or the control solution was delivered to the participant's mouth. The participant was instructed to roll the liquid around on his tongue, and after 10 seconds was given a visual cue to swallow the liquid. The liquids were delivered in sequence in each block: For instance, participants received tomato juice in one block, then the tasteless control solution, then the chocolate milk, then again the tasteless control solution. This cycle was repeated 16 times. During the imaging run, participants used a button box to indicate their subjective pleasantness of the taste stimuli on a visual rating scale ranging from + 2 (very pleasant) to − 2 (very unpleasant).

After the initial scanning, participants were taken out of the scanner and fed to satiety on one of the liquid foods. They were instructed to consume the liquid foods for their lunch and to drink as much of them as they could until they really did not want any more. The liquid food was poured into a cup and offered to the participant. Once the participant had drunk the contents of the cup, it was refilled. This was repeated a number of times until the participant was completely satiated and refused the offer of an additional cup.

To achieve a balanced design, five participants were fed to satiety on tomato juice and the other five participants were fed to satiety on the chocolate milk. Each participant was randomly allocated one of the two liquid foods for their meal and the participants were not informed in advance (until after the first imaging run) which liquid food they would be invited to consume.

Once the participants had finished their meal, the most important part of the experiment took place. They went back into the scanner and the scanning procedure was repeated exactly as before. At this point, we found that regardless of whether the participants had been fed on chocolate milk or tomato juice, they reported not liking them any more, and gave negative scores. But the same participants still liked the stimulus that they had not been fed. Importantly, it was only the participants' subjective *pleasantness* ratings that had changed, not their intensity ratings.

The changes in brain activity over the course of the experiment were correlated with the subjective pleasantness ratings for all participants. Statistical analysis revealed that a part of the mid-anterior orbitofrontal cortex was correlated with the participants' subjective experience of pleasantness. Because only the subjective pleasantness, not the intensity, ratings had changed, and the experiment was counterbalanced in terms of stimuli, this finding shows that the brain activity we recorded is not related to the pleasantness of only chocolate milk or tomato juice, but of both, and therefore to the pleasantness elicited by the combination of taste, smell, and structure of these foods.

Other studies in our laboratory and elsewhere have since found similar correlates of subjective experience of pleasure. Our studies of the subjective effects of amphetamine show that the activity in the orbitofrontal cortex also follows the ratings of the subjective experience of amphetamine. Studies from other research groups have similarly shown that such stimulants as opium, cocaine, and amphetamine (as well as sex, as shown in the following chapter) give rise to activity in the same brain regions as food, but to a stronger degree. However, this stronger activation does not necessarily mean that people would choose drugs and sex over food and drink if faced with starvation. Instead it suggests that drugs and sex are using the same reward circuits as food.

Before we return to the matter of subjective experience of pleasure in food and other stimulants, let us compare it with another type of subjective experience, pain. Pain is always defined subjectively, and it is only recently that we have gained better insight into the working of pain-relieving stimulants such as opium, and how *placebos*, which are essentially nonactive substances, can induce pain relief.

SUBJECTIVE PLACEBO

Pain scares us almost more than anything else, and incredible amounts of analgesics are consumed every day. Most of this medicine is not particularly effective in relieving pain. It even can have frightening side effects, especially in older people, who easily develop adverse symptoms such as ulcers and stomach bleeding. But there is an effective pain therapy that is without side effects, is impossible to overdose on, works for at least a third of us, and works not only for pain, but almost all other known symptoms. Although this sounds like the miracle medicines of past ages, it is a miracle that lives in all of us.

This treatment is called the *placebo effect*, and is known to bring about healing even when the treatment is complete humbug. The effect owes its name to opening words of psalm 114 (in Latin) "*Placebo Domino*...," which was used in the

Middle Ages at the Vespers for All Souls. The phenomenon was noted by the sixteenth century French essayist Michel de Montaigne, among others.

Medical studies have shown that placebo can be fairly effective against a wide variety of diseases such as heart problems, depression, Parkinson's disease, and ulcers. However, its most effective use is as a treatment for pain.

Pain is a curious subjective phenomenon that is still not fully understood. We know all too well how to inflict physical pain on others; but the same physical treatment can give rise to very different pain in different individuals (as well as pleasure in some). Pain is often without a direct physical cause. It is therefore always defined subjectively, and is hard to measure scientifically.

Clearly, therefore, this subjective experience of pain must take place in the brain, and it would be interesting to work out how placebos influence this, because such knowledge might help develop better strategies for the treatment of pain. Recently, such promise has been furthered by brain-imaging studies that give us new insights into the functional anatomy of pain. Several experiments have shown which parts of the brain are involved in different components of the experience of pain, and experiments by the Swedish neuroscientist Predrag Petrovic and colleagues have given us insights into how placebos influence our perception of pain.

One of these experiments was fairly simple, essentially consisting of comparing two warm states, one with and one without pain. Participants went through these states under the influence of opiates and placebo, letting the researchers compare participants' experience of the two warm states, but more importantly, they could also compare the differences in the participants' brains between the opiate-induced and placebo states.

The Emotional Life of Pain

The results of this placebo experiment made clear that many parts of the brain are involved in the experience of pain, but that some parts are more important than others. The main focus of many pain studies has been the anterior cingulate cortex, situated in the middle of the brain, just above the corpus callosum. Petrovic's experiment showed this brain structure to be particularly active in the placebo state.

But perhaps even more interesting was the finding that the orbitofrontal cortex was active in both the placebo and opiate-induced states This supports the findings from experiments on food and stimulants described above. The placebo experiment tells us more about which brain structures are involved in placebo for pain, indicating that there are differences in how much opiates relieve pain in different people. Other studies have shown a behavioral link between pain relief with opiates and with placebo. It looks as though the placebo effect works especially well with people who respond well to opiates.

In other words, placebo signals the brain to activate already-existing systems to combat pain and disease. So placebo is probably not just a generic mechanism, but a description of the recycling of existing brain mechanisms. When it comes to fighting illness, placebo mechanisms must be controlling parts of the immune system that would not otherwise have been activated.

This link between the brain and the immune system was called *neuropsychoimmunology* by the Danish Nobel-Prize-winning immunologist Niels Kaj Jerne, who brushed it aside as being as boring and arid as the length of the word itself. But even Nobel-Prize-winners can be wrong at times, and newer research into the placebo effect opens up a deeper understanding of the links between brain and body.

The scientific understanding of the placebo effect is still not advanced enough for systematic use. However, many of the latest findings could lead to the development of new methods of pain relief. The placebo experiment mentioned above shows a fast-working pain system that directly influences the brainstem, but one that can be modulated by other brain regions. As we learn more about this system, we may be able to develop more effective treatments.

As mentioned in several earlier chapters, we have recently gained more insights into the basic mechanisms underlying chronic pain using a technique called *deep brain stimulation*. This technique makes it possible to target deep brain regions by surgically placing an electrode directly in the brain, which can then be electrically stimulated. Deep brain stimulation has been remarkably successful in alleviating the symptoms of otherwise treatment-resistant disorders. These mainly include chronic pain, phantom pain, cluster headache, and motor disorders including Parkinson's disease, multiple sclerosis, essential tremor, dystonia, and spasmodic torticollis. Some success has also recently been reported for unipolar depression. So far the data suggests that low-frequency stimulation works particularly well for the treatment of pain, while high-frequency stimulation works best for movement disorders. For chronic pain including phantom limb pain, the most successful brain targets have been the periaqueductal gray in the brainstem and the thalamus.

We used the noninvasive neuroimaging technique of magnetoencephalography to map changes in brain activity induced by deep brain stimulation in a patient with severe phantom limb pain. When the stimulator was turned off, the patient reported significant increases in subjective pain. Corresponding significant changes in brain activity were found in a network including the mid-anterior orbitofrontal and subgenual cingulate cortices. This finding fits well with the pain-relief networks reported in the earlier placebo studies and opens the possibility that these brain regions could potentially serve as future surgical targets to relieve chronic pain.

Pain remains a basic condition of our existence, because a life without pain is very difficult and most often results in a very short life. We know this because those few people born without pain receptors often live for only a short time. For instance, without pain to tell us when a muscle has been stretched too far, we are forced constantly to give conscious attention to our movements—which is almost impossible, and the attempt leads to the attrition of the body. By contrast, normal people have a degree of pain that they must try to minimize when it becomes chronic—but which in moderation and when relieved, reminds them of its antithesis, pleasure. In some ways, placebo demonstrates that our brains let us control our own perception of pain and pleasure.

The close links between pleasure and pain are also evident in our use of stimulants. These links give rise to pain relief but also to deep pleasure, and this has been regarded with suspicion in many Western societies. In the following sections, we will look at the historical accidents that have led to some stimulants becoming stigmatized and made illegal.

PSYCHOACTIVE CULTIVATED PLANTS

The ethnobotanist Richard Evans Schultes spent 14 years gathering over 25,000 plants in the Northwestern parts of the Amazon rainforest before he became a professor at Harvard University's botanical museum. Having contracted several tropical diseases in the field, he then sent his students on large expeditions on his behalf.

Schultes always recommended that his students try any euphoriant and hallucinogenic plants they found on their field trips, believing that the individual has inviolable freedom. For a while, he became famous for helping Harvard students who had fallen foul of the law through smoking marijuana. Using a subtle taxonomic argument, Schultes would claim on the witness stand that the marijuana used by the accused was different from that which the law prohibited. The law was changed to include all sub-species of marijuana only towards the end of the 1960s, when use of euphoriant drugs in society at large rose strongly. But by then, Schultes had already become a legend at Harvard.

But why has the reputation of marijuana become so blackened over time? An increasing amount of scientific data shows that marijuana not only induces pleasure, but also has many other interesting medical attributes, especially in the area of pain relief.

The late American evolutionary biologist and writer Stephen Jay Gould has described how he used marijuana for a malignant case of stomach cancer, a disease survived by only a small and exclusive group of people. Gould belonged to this group, but at the price of a long and ruthless chemotherapy treatment that could kill the patient before it killed the cancer, particularly if the patient is forced to stop eating because of the nausea that chemotherapy invariably induces.

Although Gould did not have much faith in alternative healing, he knew he had to fight the nausea at all costs. First he tried all the legal medicine he could lay his hands on, which helped somewhat, but only before the nausea became too intense. Gould had heard that marijuana could help with the nausea, but as a somewhat atypical child of the 1960s, he hated all euphoriant drugs, and anything else that stopped the brain from functioning at its maximal capacity. But when, after much hesitation, he tried smoking marijuana after chemotherapy, the effects were strong and immediate. The nausea—and especially the paralyzing fear of nausea—disappeared, and life suddenly became tolerable again. Gould still did not enjoy the mildly intoxicating state that is a known side effect of marijuana, but he tolerated it because it was so much less an evil than the nausea.

Useful Hemp

The hemp plant and its extract marijuana have many useful medicinal attributes that also help patients suffering from multiple sclerosis, glaucoma, AIDS, depression, and other diseases.

The active ingredient in marijuana, tetrahydrocannabinol, influences the body in many ways, some of which have yet to be fully understood. Tetrahydrocannabinol has been synthesized, but this form seems to be less effective than the naturally-occurring form, which can restore the appetite of cancer patients undergoing chemotherapy, and relieve the pressure on the eyes of glaucoma sufferers, thereby improving their eyesight.

Despite these benefits, marijuana has been classified as a prohibited *narcotic* since the early 1900s. This has so stigmatized the substance that doctors and patients are often unwilling to try it, despite its incontrovertible beneficial effects.

But marijuana has been known as a remedy since ancient times. As far as we know, hemp is one of the oldest cultivated psychoactive plants in the world. In Central Asia, marijuana has been grown for more than 10,000 years. A Chinese text that is over 4,000 years old praises hemp for its beneficial effects on such ailments as malaria and arthritis. Herodotus mentions the use of hemp by the Scythians for pleasure. The plant also was widely cultivated throughout the Middle Ages; the French writer François Rabelais wrote in the 1500s about its usages to ease the pain of gout, treat burns, and cure horses of colic. At around the same time, the English writer William Turner wrote about hemp's medicinal use and quoted an earlier author on its well-known psychoactive effects.

In the 1600s, the English clergyman Robert Burton recommended marijuana as a cure for melancholia (as depression was known in those days), but it was not until the middle of the 1800s that Western medicine awoke to the plant's medical benefits.

The Irish physician William O'Shaughnessy brought medical knowledge of hemp home from India. Over the next decades, marijuana was used and subjected to close examination. It has mischievously been suggested that more was known about the medical use of marijuana in the 1800s than is known today.

But after the 1890s, interest in the hemp plant declined, due primarily to the emergence of stronger, chemically synthesized drugs. However, the side effects of the hemp plant are mild, if any, whereas it eventually became apparent that the stronger drugs caused strong side effects, such as bleeding ulcers.

In 1937 the United States banned marijuana. The law was intended to stop its recreational use, and can be regarded as an example of the puritanical streak in American society (as shown earlier by the 1920–1933 prohibition of alcohol). Although the law may not have been designed to prohibit the medical use of marijuana, this quickly became its effect when doctors could no longer easily obtain legal supplies for treatment.

During the 1960s, articles on the medicinal use of marijuana appeared largely in magazines such as *Playboy*, and marijuana became associated with its widespread use as a recreational drug by a new generation of baby boomers experimenting with alternative ways of living. The following decade saw the introduction of the "war on drugs," which classified drugs in four groups. This led to an intense debate about the category marijuana should be placed in, a debate that remains to this day. At the same time, following strong pressure from patients and doctors, some American states started discreetly permitting medicinal use of marijuana.

Today, interest in the medical properties of marijuana is being revived all over the world. Scientific studies consistently show that marijuana is far less harmful than, for example, alcohol. In stark contrast to alcohol, marijuana's medical properties can help patients with certain medical conditions. Yet the continuing stigma attached to marijuana means that patients who could benefit from it are suffering needlessly.

THE PLANT OF IMMORTALITY

Marijuana is not the only cultural plant to have been stigmatized throughout the ages. Another highly controversial one is the coca plant, the use of which is closely intertwined with the history of suffering in South America. How did such a small shrub become the object of such adoration and condemnation?

The Western world has seen the coca plant alternately as an incredible stimulant capable of curing everything, or as evil incarnate. Today, the political powers have settled on the latter. They press for complete eradication of the plant because cocaine can be extracted from its leaves. On the other side of this divide are the indigenous people of South America who have used the coca plant as an integral part of their unique cultures for thousands of years. They have worshipped it as the plant of immortality. Many chew coca leaves to endure hunger, thirst, and inhumane working conditions.

The coca plant is a strong bush that can adapt to different climates. Its leaves are rich in vitamins and minerals.

One hundred grams of coca leaves contain more nutrients than the total daily recommendation in the United States. The leaves are therefore a necessary supplement to the diet in South America, which is traditionally poor in both nutrients and milk products. In Bolivia, coca is used as an additive in products that range from toothpaste to tea. In addition, coca leaves have a stimulating and appetizing effect.

In South America, especially in the highlands of the Andes, millions of people chew coca leaves with alkalines such as volcanic ash. This chewing lets nutrients from the leaves enter the bloodstream slowly through the stomach. For many, the chewing is part of a daily routine, just as we drink tea and coffee in the West, both for their taste and to absorb the psychoactive variants of caffeine. The harsh conditions of the highlands have encouraged coca chewing, which strengthens and nourishes while rarely causing mental illness, only a nicotine-like dependence.

The Sacred Plant of the Incas

Like many other indigenous people in South America, the Incas worshipped the coca plant. For them, the coca plant was the most sacred of all plants, and the coca leaves were a divine manifestation of the immortal soul. The great Inca Empire was bristling with large coca plantations and everyone used the stimulating leaves. Chewing coca leaves was a part of religious ceremonies, and the future was read in the leaves. The ill and dying were given coca leaves, because the taste of coca at death was the only way to a good afterlife. The vast Inca Empire also used coca leaves to maintain the strength of its armies and all those who had to travel its enormous empire.

When the Spaniards came to South America in the 1500s, they brought with them a holy mission to spread the "one true faith"—and an unquenchable thirst for gold. They soon started giving coca leaves to the enslaved indigenous mine workers to maximize their performance. The Spaniards took over the coca plantations. Although the Roman Catholic Church banned the plant on the grounds that it helped sustain the heathen beliefs of the indigenous population, too many of the Spanish colonialists were by then making fortunes from selling the plant, and from maintaining the inhuman output of the mines. Furthermore, much of the Church's income in South America came from tax on the coca plant, so the ban was raised, allowing the coca plant to be cultivated and sold but prohibiting its use in religious ceremonies on pain of death.

This maelstrom of Spanish conquest, with its suffering, death, high taxes, and relentless work, served to enlarge and extend the cultural identity of the indigenous population which became known as *rukuna*, the people. Chewing coca leaves came to be seen as the purest expression of that identity. Thus the Spanish conquest indirectly contributed to the survival of indigenous cultural identities, which persists to this day.

Papal Blessing

Towards the end of the 1800s, North America and Europe discovered the stimulating effects of the coca plant. Within a few decades, it went from being a praised stimulant preferred by popes to a modern curse. First it became popular to use coca plant extracts as a stimulant in different products. A red wine called *Vin Mariani*, containing coca, was marketed as a tonic to refresh both body and soul. It became such a success that Pope Leo XIII gave it a gold medal for inspiring courage and strength in the work of priests.

Coca leaves also were used in lozenges and soft drinks, including Coca Cola, which quickly found a large market. It was sold as a form of spring water that strengthened the poor man's soul. Cocaine was removed from the product in 1906, but nutrients from the coca leaves are still included as important "natural taste ingredients."

In 1860, pure cocaine was produced from coca leaves for the first time. Among others, Sigmund Freud was enthusiastic about the drug. He saw the psychoactive drug cocaine as a miracle cure—for morphine addiction and alcoholism, for example. But it soon became clear that the cure could be as bad as the disease, because cocaine causes different effects than coca. Cocaine influences the brain by activating mechanisms that are less strongly activated by other rewards such as food intake. When cocaine is taken in small doses, it elicits a feeling of well being, strength, and mental vigor. But taken in larger quantities, and with repeated use over extended periods, it can lead to depression, mental disturbances, anxiety, sleep problems, and paranoia. Although it is not nearly as addictive as, say, heroin, cocaine nevertheless almost always causes dependency.

Over the years, more and more restrictions were imposed on cocaine. In 1922, it was classified as a narcotic drug, with the attached stigma of corruption and evil. In 1950, the United Nations tried to eradicate the coca plant by recommending a global ban on it. The thinking behind this was that the coca plant caused physical, moral, economic, and social problems. The proposal was strongly protested by Peru and Bolivia, who argued that the eradication of the plant would cause immeasurable damage to their population. However, 11 years later, economic pressures forced these countries to sign the agreement.

During the 1960s, cocaine became increasingly popular as a recreational drug in the West. In a repeat of events 100 years earlier, it was first seen as harmless, and its use became widespread. But as with other types of drugs, abuse of this one leads to serious problems for the individual, so the West, particularly the United States, has sought to eradicate the coca plant. This is similar to the attempts to eradicate the opium poppy (and thereby heroin) in Afghanistan and other countries.

But once again, it is worth asking whether eradication of the coca plant would really solve our drug problem. Cocaine is linked to the coca plant and would presumably disappear if the plant were eradicated. But would this eradicate the human desire for drugs? A more likely scenario is that synthetically produced drugs would take over the role of cocaine on the global market.

Perhaps destroying the coca plant would destroy only the vestiges of ancient cultures in South America, which may well include the soul of the indigenous peoples. So some may well question the wisdom of doing so.

BRAINY SOLUTIONS?

There are no easy solutions to our dependence on stimulants such as marijuana, cocaine, amphetamine, and heroin. The same is obviously true for sex, and also for the problems caused by our somewhat overlooked, but at least as serious, addiction to sugary, fatty, and salty foods. Obesity and eating disorders constitute a hidden epidemic causing serious health problems that need addressing. However, stimulants such as cocaine are hooked into the brain's reward mechanisms, and users reach selective satiation with them with much greater difficulty. Exactly, because these stimulants all use the same learning mechanisms that are essential to keep

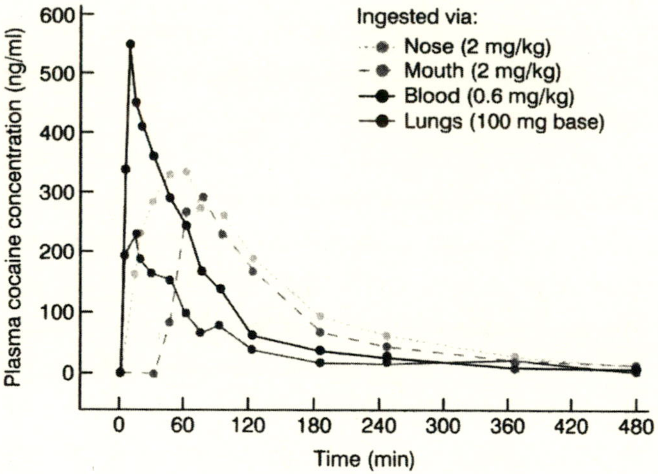

Figure 9.2 The effects of stimulants. The same amount of a stimulant can have very different effects depending on which method is used. The figure shows how the plasma concentration of cocaine changes over time. The fastest and most effective method is through injection in the blood stream (black line), where the maximal effect is obtained after a few minutes. Smoking is almost as quick but does not affect the plasma concentration as much (dark gray). Taking cocaine through the nose leads to maximal effects after almost 60 minutes (light stippled gray) compared to almost 90 minutes when eaten (medium stippled gray).

us alive, it is hard to find appropriate strategies to break this dependency (Figure 9.2).

Prohibition and criminalization are clearly not working; many drug-related problems in the West are intimately connected to social prohibitions, because many people are forced into crime in order to maintain their drug addiction. Some people who want to legalize drugs cite examples of heroin addicts who hold down normal jobs—as long as their habit does not cost so much that it drags them into crime. But we lack solid data to decide whether legalization is realistic, and we need an informed debate about whether drug addiction can acceptably coexist with a normal existence.

We also have to realize that drug criminalization has resulted in this fact, at least 8% of the money circulating in the world has direct connections to the drug trade. Furthermore, enormous amounts are spent imprisoning people on drug-related charges, and reintegrating drug felons back into society.

Perhaps we have to learn to accept that the human brain makes us disproportionately interested in pleasure. Desire for pleasure is part of human nature, and criminalizing it does not seem to work. What certainly does not work is dishonest campaigns about the malignant effects of drugs. Drugs do elicit desires and pleasure. Stating anything else is misleading and counterproductive, so reliable information should let young people learn how to manage these desires and pleasures.

It is also important to address the social element in drug addiction. Initially, drugs are often taken as part of a collective experience, as the Kofán Indians (from whom Schultes learned so much about the plants of Ecuador and Colombia) take them. Yet it is the antisocial effects of drug-taking that are wreaking havoc on society.

There are no easy solutions to control drug addiction. As mentioned in other chapters, moderation and variation are the most important principles for all desires and pleasures. Recognizing this might help avoid the consequences of drug addiction that threaten to undermine both our health systems and the wider society.

● ● ● HAPPINESS LESSONS

Contrary to official dogma, natural forms of some drugs can be beneficial, depending on circumstances and personalities involved, and always assuming moderation. Evaluate these dispassionately rather than using flawed or uninformed assumptions.

Our reactions to food developed to facilitate survival in environments of scarcity. Don't blindly follow food desires into overindulgence. Once again, variation and moderation are key.

FURTHER READING

Indigenous people have remarkable insight into the efficacy of plants—as studied in the science of ethnobotany. Two excellent books should be recommended, Balick, M. J. & Cox, P. A. (1996), *Plants, People, and Culture. The Science of Ethnobotany.* New York, NY: W H Freeman. Davis, W. (1996) *One River.*

Explorations and Discoveries in the Amazon Rain Forest. New York, NY: Simon & Schuster.

More interesting knowledge about marijuana can be gathered from the following books: Grinspoon, L. & Bakalar, J. B. (1997). *Marihuana, the Forbidden Medicine.* New Haven: Yale Unversity Press. Iversen, L. L. (2007). *The Science of Marijuana.*2nd edition. Oxford: Oxford University Press.

The global history of drugs is described in, Davenport-Hines, R. (2002). *The Pursuit of Oblivion: A Global History of Narcotics.* London: W.W. Norton.

10

SEX

Reproducing Love

Chastity. The most unnatural of the sexual perversions

Aldous Huxley (1894–1963)

Travelling in China in the early 1990s, I witnessed one of life's more monumental events. It arrived entirely unexpected during an otherwise depressing visit to a run-down zoo that resembled a cramped prison populated by catatonic panda bears. As we fought our way through the crowds with their nauseating reams of candy floss, suddenly an even more cloying, almost unbearable smell hit my nostrils. Almost against my will, I followed the smell to a metal fence with large bales of straw, but I was completely unprepared for what was to follow.

Just in front of us, two elephants emerged and gave us a full view of the events about to unfold. One of the elephants was rather larger than the other and the former's man-sized erect sexual organ left little doubt with regard to gender. The smaller female elephant was waiting passively with her back to the male elephant, who was flapping his ears while making rutting calls. Then he lifted his forelegs unto her back and lay his long trunk along her back and head. With his weight on his hind legs and his penis partly folded in the shape of a horizontal "s," he tried to find the entrance and succeeded after a few attempts. The female elephant passively received his thrusting for about 1 minute, after which the male elephant slid out and left her standing.

The female started to utter a series of deep sounds that grew and diminished in volume over and over again. Then the sounds were amplified by a series of calls from other female elephants standing in a nearby enclosure. The female elephant started flapping her ears and trumpeting passionately, to which the other females responded with their own trumpet calls.

I was flabbergasted. The events had lasted only about 5 minutes, but I had never before and have not since witnessed that deep rumbling or trembling. It was the majestic character of the moment that demonstrated the deep intensity that sex can trigger in large, intelligent animals such as elephants. Moreover, somewhat more prosaically, research has since demonstrated that the deep trembling I witnessed is likely to have come from the infrasound used by elephants for communication.

● MISSIONARY COUSINS

Reproduction and associated behavior are crucial for the survival of all animals. But not all acts of reproduction are as monumental as those of elephants. It is not surprising that much of animal behavior is about getting into a position where reproduction becomes possible. The brain reward for successful sexual behavior is so strong that this behavior is given priority at the expense of almost all other forms of behavior except for eating and sleeping.

Humans are not the only or most advanced animal with the ability to separate procreation and reproduction. We appear to share this ability with our primate cousin, the bonobo. It is a relatively rare primate species with a behavior that lives up to the old slogan of "*make love, not war*" to a greater extent than the most emancipated hippies. The bonobo ape is one of the last great primates discovered. In 1929, the German physiologist Ernst Schwarz discovered that what he had mistaken for a juvenile chimpanzee was in fact a fully grown ape. It became clear that it was a new species.

The new species was given the Latin name *Pan paniscus*. Sometimes, it is also called the *pygmy-chimpanzee*, which is misleading in terms of size, that name derives from the fact that like the pygmies, the bonobos have their home in the rainforest south of the Zaire (Congo) river.

Solving Conflict with Sex

The average life span of a bonobo is still unknown but probably comparable to that of the chimpanzee, around 40 years in the wild. The bonobo is nursed by its mother until it is about 5 years old, and is fully grown at 15 years.

Fresh fruit is the primary sustenance for both the bonobo and the chimpanzee. Chimpanzees fill their need for animal protein by eating smaller monkeys that they capture and kill. In contrast, bonobos appear to fill this need by eating a special plant, so it is rare to see bonobos catching smaller monkeys to eat them. Instead, they appear to catch them just to play with them. Where chimpanzees use tools to obtain food, this type of behavior has not been observed in bonobos in the wild. Captured bonobos are adept at using tools, so the lack of tool use in the wild is probably more likely linked to the abundance of easily accessible food.

For better or worse, studies of chimpanzee behavior both in zoos and in the wild have shown a close relationship to humans. Like humans, chimpanzees use tools, cooperative hunting, and primitive warfare. So for many years, it was assumed that chimpanzees were the best living model to our ancestors. Because the male chimpanzee is totally dominant, many saw this as an expression of the natural order.

But the bonobos diverge radically from this notion. Bonobo society is controlled by the females. It is peaceful compared to chimpanzee society, in which researchers have documented infanticide and brutal warlike behavior.

The secret of the peaceful bonobo society appears to rest with their sexual behavior; in their society, sex is used to solve conflicts. Food or anything else that awakens the interest of bonobos will elicit sexual contact between the involved parties. This way bonobos appear to use sex to divert attention from and tone down the aggression present in chimpanzees and other primates.

This sexual contact is often short-lived and remarkably varied. As observed in 1954 by Austrian zoologists Eduard Tratz and Heinz Heck, bonobos use face-to-face copulation, unlike chimpanzees who almost always copulate like dogs. In earlier times, some researchers regarded face-to-face copulation as a unique human trait. Some even went as far as to propose that this "advanced" form of sexual contact, named the missionary position, was a cultural phenomenon that should be taught to so-called primitive humans. It was initially controversial that bonobos, with their human-like anatomy in which vulva and clitoris is oriented forward, would use this position naturally, and quite often—in one of three matings in the wild.

It appears that most sexual variations known in humans are used by bonobos. In addition, bonobos have added a number of variations such as genito-genital rubbing between females, which appears to induce an orgasm-like state. Even orgasm is not a uniquely human state, as is known from studies of rhesus monkey and others species. The average sexual contact between bonobos is around 13 seconds, which is somewhat quick even compared to human standards.

In addition to decidedly sexual behavior, adult bonobos exhibit other behaviors that are best classified as erotic because they may not lead to reproduction. An example is the widespread practice of mouth-to-mouth kissing, most often involving the tongue. "French kissing" is not found in chimpanzees, whose kissing is almost platonic. One newly appointed zookeeper who was used to working with chimpanzees therefore accepted a kiss from a male bonobo. He was subsequently very surprised to experience the whole tongue of the bonobo in his mouth.

However, it would be wrong to draw the conclusion that bonobos as a species are pathologically fixated on sex and sexually deranged. Instead, sex is a recreational part of everyday bonobo life, just as is the case with most humans. Sex is not used all the time, but occasionally.

Mother and Son

This leads back to the female status in bonobo society. Both chimpanzees and bonobos live in groups in which the male apes remain in their original group and the females migrate. Male chimpanzees form strong bonds among themselves for hunting and protecting their territory. But female chimpanzees do not create particularly strong bonds either to other females or to one particular male. Therefore female chimpanzees are often marginalized in the social hierarchy. This is in striking contrast to female bonobos, who create close social bonds both with other females and with their own sons.

The male chimpanzee's social status depends critically on the alliances he is able to form with other males from the group. In contrast, the status of a male bonobo depends on the position of his mother in bonobo society. So the mother–son relationship is decisive for determining social status, and mother and son remain together for life.

Bonobo society is not only centered on females, but also dominated by them. Whereas male chimpanzees always get first access to food, it is always the dominant group of bonobo females who eat first (after some genito-genital rubbing). Only then is the male bonobo allowed to eat. It has also been observed how a group of female bonobos will gang up on a male bonobo as a way of pacifying him.

More contrast to chimpanzees: Female bonobos almost always have pink genital swellings, which signal that female is sexually available. In this way, females hide their ovulations and thus when they can be inseminated. That means that the male bonobo is unable to guess who is among his offspring, which probably avoids the infanticide observed in chimpanzees by the English primatologist Jane Goodall.

THROUGH A LOOKING GLASS

Studies of groups of bonobos and chimpanzees have added to our understanding of the complex social patterns that exist among our distant relatives. These ingenious social patterns are constantly changing and if anything, bear witness to the advanced intelligence of the apes. The clever use of tools in chimpanzees and their remarkable ability for solving even complicated problems are well-documented. But convincing evidence for full-blown language has not been demonstrated, so researchers have refused to recognize the intelligence of chimpanzees as comparable to anything but that of a young child. But studies of bonobos seem to demonstrate that they may have the ability for protolanguage. The American primatologist Sue Savage-Rumbaugh has for many years used lexigrams to show how the bonobo Kanzi masters language. Whether Kanzi possesses human-like language remains a subject for academic discussions, but it is clear that he can both understand and produce language to an impressive degree.

Kanzi typically constructs sentences with two or three elements, which is comparable to a 2- or 3-year-old human child before language development starts in earnest. The sentences show a certain order that could point towards an underlying grammatical structure. Of course this is highly controversial among linguists who would argue that grammar is the foundation for natural language.

Kanzi's understanding of language is possibly even more impressive than his production of it. Many animal species appear to be able to guess what is being said from contextual cues, including vocal pitch and body language. To avoid such charges, Kanzi is made to listen through headphones to the sentences from a person in another room. Kanzi does not hesitate to take the correct picture from a pile of pictures, and to connect different objects. If Savage-Rumbaugh asks him to "put the pines in the fridge," Kanzi will do so.

A central question is to what extent language understanding corresponds to production. At the very least, understanding must demand active listening to what are often only incomplete language fragments followed by attempts to understand and reconstruct meaning. A good example is the sentence "wreck a nice beach," which can easily be misheard as "recognize speech."

In addition, these higher apes also appear to have the ability for self-recognition. As mentioned earlier, American psychologist Gordon Gallup invented a test that has demonstrated that both bonobos and chimpanzees can recognize themselves in a mirror. This indicates that they may be self-conscious to a degree that resembles our own. In contrast, the gorilla does not show signs of mirror self-recognition.

Many other signs in bonobos and chimpanzees indicate that their intelligence is first and foremost of a social nature.

Their brains resemble the human brain. Some researchers have even proposed that the behavior of bonobos may resemble one of our early ancestors. *Australopithecus afarensis*. The members of this species are likely to have lived in trees, but like the bonobo, they sometimes walked on two legs, as shown by the discovery of the remains of footprints south of the Olduvai gorge in Tanzania.

Through the study of bonobos, we may have a unique possibility to understand our evolutionary past and perhaps even come to terms with the sexuality driving our behavior. Unfortunately, however, with the ongoing hostilities in Congo, the prospects for the long-term survival of this fascinating ape are slim, and will require active intervention on their behalf.

SEX, LIES, AND SCIENCE

Human behavior is perhaps best differentiated from that of other animals by the complexity of human life. In addition, human language lets us to talk about what we do when the lights are turned off. But exactly because of this incontrovertible complexity of human behavior, the natural variation is also great. Human sexual behavior remains shrouded in mystery.

This does not prevent almost all daily newspapers and magazines from having a column dedicated to sex and its problems. A recent selection of these included such more or less reliable findings that occasional masturbation is harmless, homosexuality is common, vaginal orgasms are rare, and both having a lot and having no sex is not uncommon.

We owe the credit for many of these well-documented facts to American sex researcher Alfred C. Kinsey, who started his career collecting wasps and continued to build the largest collection of sex material in the world. This collection included 18,500 interviews with men and women about their sexual habits, as well as footage of more than 2000 male ejaculations and hundreds of films of mating behavior in rats, horses, pigeons and pigs.

The results of Kinsey's scientific investigations of the human sexuality were published in two monumental volumes in 1948 and 1953. These investigations changed our understanding of human sexuality. Yet, as is often the case with all radical insights. Kinsey's findings provoked great controversy.

Most controversial was the statistic that 37% of all men have homosexual experiences, that 10% of men have homosexual relationships lasting longer than 3 years, and that 4% are exclusively homosexual throughout life. Kinsey therefore found it counterproductive that homosexuality was seen as a crime in most American states at the time of his studies. However, such progressive ideas were not shared by certain segments of the American society in the 1950s, so his ideas and methods came under attack.

Sex Interviews

Like other scientific researchers of human sexuality, Kinsey used interviews to obtain information. But the problem with interviews, or any form of conversation, is that lying is difficult to detect—and that people often lie about taboo subjects such as sex. Other problems, such as the interviewer posing leading questions, may also limit the utility of the information obtained.

Kinsey tried to minimize these problems by developing a special method. He always used face-to-face interviews, and he bombarded people with questions and control questions to minimize their possibility for lying or hiding facts. In addition, Kinsey would ask the same questions in slightly different ways, and the answers were coded on a single sheet. When Kinsey had perfected his method, he spent up to a whole year training his colleagues. This is in stark contrast to other, later studies that have often used simple questionnaires and brief training courses, and were sometimes even conducted over the phone.

A potential criticism with scientific studies can be that the groups studied are not representative of the general population. Some of the attacks on Kinsey's methods pointed out that because he had interviewed prison inmates, this had distorted the statistics for homosexuality. However, subsequent reanalysis showed that the statistics were not significantly different when the prison group was removed.

Trisexuality, Animal Sex, and Monomania

Until recently, most of Kinsey's overall scientific conclusions were not called into question by other scientists. But a very critical biography of Kinsey was published in 1997 by James Jones, who argued that Kinsey's own homosexuality and sadomasochistic tendencies had perverted his data and methods enough that his conclusions should be called into question. This was the first time the general public was given detailed access to information about Kinsey's sexuality, and it quickly mounted a storm, perhaps reflecting the homophobia that still exists in society.

Although Kinsey defined himself as bisexual, he was perhaps best described as "trisexual," someone who would try anything. But it is difficult to see how this can be held against him. Rather it would seem important for a sex researcher to help reveal the large variation in sexual habits.

Why should it change our views of Kinsey's measurements of penis size that Kinsey apparently was well endowed? Although various independent scientific studies have found that the average size ranges from 12.8 to 15.4 centimeters (about 5 to 6 inches), this variation is probably more linked to the fact that measuring penises is an inexact science with erect and nonerect states and a wide natural variation from small (3 centimeters or about 1 inch) to large (35 centimeters or about thirteen and three-quarter inches).

Other more recent studies of homosexuality have found a slightly different incidence than Kinsey did. But this does not change the fact that *all* serious sex studies have found that homosexuality is naturally occurring among both men and women, so it would seem prudent not to criminalize this behavior.

Kinsey's findings do not pertain only to homosexuality, but offer an insightful, thorough and nuanced portrait of human sexuality in general. Yet his honesty challenged the preconceptions of many. For example, his data showed that at least 17% of American men who worked on farms had had sex to orgasm with animals ranging from dogs, pigs, cows and sheep to bulls and chickens. Kinsey believed that the real number was probably double that. As with other solitary activities, animal sex was most common among men with a higher education.

Rather than condemn these people, Kinsey wrote with great empathy of the strong feelings bordering on passion that many of these boys and young men showed towards their livestock. Because he was trained as a zoologist, he may have wanted to show how humans are closely linked to other animals.

But Kinsey did not legitimize all sexual behavior. He interviewed rapists and pedophiles in prisons for a book he planned on sex crimes. Although he always tried to remain open to the variation of human sexual behavior, he was shaken to his core by the criminals' revelations, especially the fact that most of them planned to continue their dark deeds upon release. Kinsey's considered opinion was that these people should remain in prison with the key thrown away.

Like many other scientists with radical ideas, Kinsey showed an almost zealous determination that made collaboration difficult. There is little doubt that Kinsey exhibited monomania in his scientific mission to study and disseminate the knowledge of human sexuality. And it is likely that Kinsey was rather devoid of humor and haunted by his own demons. His studies were certainly not without faults, and some of his conclusions have to be carefully evaluated. However, this is normal for scientific enquiry and does not change the fact that Kinsey was a pioneer whose comprehensive studies revolutionized our understanding of human sexuality.

Despite the detailed scientific studies of Kinsey and other later sexologists, our knowledge of human sexuality is still imperfect. It is also almost certainly skewed, both because people tell lies and because, like much other human behavior, our sexual behaviors change over time. But between the small, large, and statistical lies about human sexuality, it is possible to discern the contours of a strange animal that habitually uses sex for much more than reproduction.

BRAIN SEX

The American sex symbol Mae West, known for her preference for recreational sex, is said to have been asked to point out the largest erogenous zone in humans. The journalist was probably taken by surprise when West immediately pointed to her brain. But of course her answer is correct. The brain is the epicenter of our subjective experiences, including sexual ones. The exploration of the sexual brain is still in its infancy because it is hard to get funding and ethical permission for it. However, some interesting findings have emerged—primarily from patients and recently from brain scanning.

Let us start with the man who claims to experience orgasms in his foot. To understand this somewhat bizarre condition, we have to make a detour to the apparently absurd situation of patients complaining of having pain in a missing limb. Many patients who undergo amputation will suffer from strong phantom pains. First described in 1871 by the English doctor Silas Weir Mitchell, this is a serious problem, because how can one cure pain in a nonexistent limb?

The fundamental function of the brain is to construct and attach meaning to events. This meaning can change radically over a short time. The following experiment is a striking example of how malleable our body image is. All you need to conduct it is a scarf and two helpers (let us call them Maya and Laura). Blindfold yourself with the scarf and seat yourself on a chair behind Maya. Tell Laura to guide the index finger of your right hand to Maya's nose. With the same finger, repeatedly and unpredictably stroke and tap Maya's nose, as if you were using Morse code. At the same time, ask Laura to stroke and tap *your* nose in exactly the same way with the index finger of her left hand. The strokes and taps on Maya's and your nose must be completely synchronous.

If the experiment is carried out correctly, after 30 to 40 seconds, you will start to experience the strange illusion of having a nose the size of Pinocchio's. The more random and unpredictable the movements, the stronger the illusion will be. It is a striking example of how quickly the brain constructs meaning on the basis of the information present.

As in the experiment described above, we can experience conflicts with what we logically know to be true. Characteristically, the brain tries to avoid these conflicts, in order to help us navigate our complex environment. However, at times this avoidance creates absurd situations. For example, consider neurological patients suffering from neglect disorders who consistently deny the existence of all objects in one half of their visual field—including in their own body.

THE WHOLE ARM

Numerous medical strategies for curing chronic pain have been tried for many years. For example, with pain in a phantom hand, further amputation was attempted, first up to the elbow and sometimes even as far up as the shoulder. When this did not work (as it rarely does), nerves were removed from the spinal cord. In some cases, even surgical intervention in the brain was tried. All too often these treatments were ineffective, and had many unpleasant side effects.

Consequently, scientists became unwilling to accept phantom pains as a real physiological disorder. Instead, some neo-Freudian theoreticians saw them as repressed wishes for lost body parts. This was more or less the situation when the Indian neurologist Vilayanur Ramachandran came up with a clever experiment.

Vision processing uses approximately half the cortex by some estimates, and has a controlling impact on our cognitive capacities. Many patients report strong pains especially in a phantom hand, which they often feel to be agonizingly clenched. So Ramachandran had a special *mirror box* made. When one hand is inserted into this box, it creates the illusion of two hands (that is, the real and the nonexistent hands). The missing hand seems to have magically returned. The chronic pain can sometimes be alleviated by asking the patient to open and close both hands in the mirror box. In one case, the mirror box not only cured the pain, but even amputated the phantom hand.

It should be mentioned that deep brain stimulation is probably the most effective therapy for chronic phantom limb pain. We will return to this effective surgical procedure, which involves inserting an electrode deep in the brain and connecting the electrode with a battery to supply repetitive burst of electricity to the targeted brain region. Deep brain stimulation of the periaquaductal gray and the ventrolateral thalamus can provide effective pain relief, although the mechanisms of the action are not yet fully understood. Some insights came to light recently when we were the first team in the world to use magnetoencephalography to record the whole brain responses when turning deep brain stimulation on and off for chronic phantom limb pain. We found that regions of the orbitofrontal and subgenual cingulate cortices were associated with the pain relief. We have also found similar regions active for pleasure. The results would thus suggest that pleasure and pain relief may use some of the same mechanisms.

This does not explain either phantom pains or orgasms in feet. In order to understand this, we need another look at the pioneering research by the American neurosurgeon Wilder Penfield in the 1950s. This research on awake epileptic patients demonstrated how the body is represented as maps in the cortex of the brain. These maps do not reflect the true proportions of the body; they are distorted. For instance, the face and genitals occupy a greater area in the brain than the elbow and toes do; we find the area for the hand, not the upper body, next to the area for the face; and we find the area for the feet, not the thighs, next to area for the genitals.

Now, what if part of the brain area for the hand were taken over by a neighboring area, in this case the face? In that case, stimulation of parts of the face should be felt in the amputated hand. This is exactly what was found. An amputee's whole hand could be found on her chin; not only could she feel needle pricks and a wet cotton swab there, but she *also* felt them in her nonexistent hand.

The reorganization in the adult brain was demonstrated to a level that many had not thought possible. Neighboring areas in the brain can overtake the functions of even a large area. Analogous effects have since been found in other animals as well as in human violinists, who use a larger part of cortex than normal subjects to represent hands and fingers.

Note that this reorganization is unlikely to depend on the formation of new neurons, because conventional wisdom contends that no new neurons are formed after birth. Although research has recently shown that this is not always the case—for example, new neurons are being formed in the hippocampus—this happens at a rate that is much less than that of neural cell death. Instead, the reorganization in relation to phantom limbs is more likely to depend on the reuse of existing connections.

So bizarre phenomena such foot orgasms and foot fetishism may be explained by the fact that the brain area for the genitals is next to the feet. But is the orgasm really to be found in the genitals or somewhere else?

SEX IN THE SCANNER

An IgNobel-Prize-winning experiment on sexual intercourse in a whole-body magnetic resonance scanner was published in the Christmas issue of the *British Medical Journal.* The IgNobel Prize is given to research "that makes people laugh and then *think.*" The study was carried out in Holland by

Willibrord Schultz and colleagues with a total of 13 experimental copulations by eight couples and sexual arousal in three single women. Because these scanners were designed for only one person, club members have to have a certain physiognomy and acrobatic abilities.

Despite the cramped conditions, the nine women reported orgasms, which they, however, rated as superficial. The experiments did not investigate the brain activity in the participants, but only the physiology, which was so difficult for the men that they were given potency enhancers.

It was the first time that researchers were able to peer inside the human body during intercourse; they found that in the missionary position, the penis has the shape of a boomerang. A third of its length consists of the root of the penis, so that the average penis including the root was all of 22 centimeters (8.7 inches) in the experiments.

This discovery was in contrast to previous anatomical drawings by Leonardo da Vinci in 1493 of a straight penis during intercourse or the "s"-shape drawn by R.S. Kendall in 1933. It was also found that the size of the female uterus did not appear to change with sexual excitement, which is at odds with the original findings by Masters and Johnson who, using a manual method, found between 50 to 100% increases of the uterus 20 minutes after orgasm. These results were thought to be due to increased blood flow, but it is now more likely to have been due to imprecise measurements.

Brain scanning of sexual excitement and orgasm is remarkably rare. Of course there are technical problems with such studies, such as the ability to keep one's head still during the experiment. But such problems are not so insurmountable that they can explain why there are so few studies. The sexual instinct would appear to be taboo to a degree that surpasses even drug studies, of which many more exist.

It was not until the end of 2003 that an interesting study of the activity in the male brain during orgasm was published; that was followed by a study of female orgasm in 2006. In 1985, scientists had tried using electroencephalography (EEG) to uncover the effects of male masturbation, but surprisingly there were no significant changes in activity. Another study was published in 1994 by a Finnish group using single photon emission computed tomography (SPECT) that found that orgasm is related to less activity in the whole brain, but more activity in the right prefrontal cortex. Unfortunately, the spatial resolution of SPECT is limited, and it is therefore difficult to evaluate these findings.

The Dutch neurologist Janniko Georgiadis and colleagues used positron emission tomography (PET) scanning to minimize the problems with orgasm-induced movement and found increased blood flow in many parts of the male brain when comparing orgasm with only sexual excitement. The strongest activity was found deep in the brainstem in the ventral tegmentum, which is closely linked to dopamine release. Similar activity has been found in experiments using rewards both natural, such as food, and artificial, such as heroin. Dopamine release appears to be linked to rewarding behavior such as ejaculation, in this instance. Other areas showing increased activity included the mid-anterior orbitofrontal cortex, anterior insula, and cerebellum, which are involved in the regulation of emotional state and learning of motor responses. The researchers also found less blood flow in the amygdala and entorhinal cortex in orgasm, with similar responses in the amygdala having been found in studies on cocaine.

The female orgasm has also recently been studied with PET by the same group of researchers. Although male orgasm is directly linked with reproduction through ejaculation, female orgasm does not serve a direct reproductive role. However, it has been proposed to serve a role for sperm retention and for attachment. In the experiment, heterosexual women achieved their orgasms through clitoral stimulation from their male partner, and their level of arousal was measured both by verbal ratings and with a rectal probe that measures rectal pressure variability. Compared to rest, the orgasm was linked to decreased activity in left mid-anterior orbitofrontal cortex, inferior temporal gyrus, and the anterior temporal pole. The results fit well with the proposed role of the orbitofrontal cortex as a mediator for subjective hedonic experience. The women's level of sexual arousal also was measured and found to correlate with activity in the medial ventral midbrain and the caudate nucleus. So these measures of desire were found to correlate with brain regions that have been implicated in the release of dopamine. Overall, the results would seem to support the distinction between separate brain regions implicated in wanting and liking.

There also have been a couple of studies of sexual excitement related to erotic images. The results are difficult to interpret because they do not include objective measurements of the sexual arousal. One study purports to have shown gender differences in brain activity when the participants were shown identical erotic images. Specifically, more activity was found in the amygdala and hypothalamus in men than in women. It is difficult to interpret such results because they can have many competing causes related specifically to the experimental setup and methods. More generally, it is also doubtful to what extent it is possible to distinguish between male and female brains.

Humans are not the only animals who find erotic images so desirable that some are willing to pay to watch them. The American neuroscientist Michael Platt and his colleagues found that male rhesus monkeys will "pay" considerable amounts of fruit juice to watch the red hindquarters of female monkeys. The monkeys also will pay to watch images of high-ranking monkeys, but they have to be paid to watch lower-ranking monkeys. This is also true for high-ranking monkeys, suggesting that for all the monkeys, the social dominance hierarchy is as important as sex. How the brain deals with social relations is a critical aspect of understanding human behavior.

EINAR WHO BECAME LILI

Some cultures have more than just two genders. In addition to the categories for male and female, these cultures recognize categories of in-betweens. Some people feel that they are born in the wrong body, and it has become possible for them to change their gender. In 1930 in Germany, the Danish artist Einar Wegener was the first person to have a sex-change operation, and eventually became Lili Elbe. Lili fell in love with her German surgeon Magnus Hirschfeld. It is not known if her love was reciprocated, but we do know that Hirschfeld convinced her to have an ovaries transplant to try to become a "true" woman. Unfortunately, the operation was too complicated for Hirschfeld, and Lili bled to death during the operation. Lili Elbe was buried in Dresden in 1931.

The first sex-change operation in the U.S. was carried out in 1952. Even today, the operation is not without risk, but many choose it over living in the wrong body.

The development of the body is the product of the genetic material developed from the fusion of spermatozoa and ovum. Sex, or sexual reproduction as it is also known, is one of evolution's more clever solutions to the problem of propagating genes containing errors. The advantage of sex is that it blends genetic material from parents, thus often avoiding potentially fatal genetic errors.

Men and women have different complementary reproduction organs (penis and vagina) and different secondary sexual characteristics. Men have testicles and more bodily hair than women, who have larger breasts and bottoms. Relatively rare cases can be found of humans, known as hermaphrodites, who have genitals that are neither penis nor vagina, but in-between.

The differences between men and women already start to develop in utero. There is considerable scientific evidence that, in contrast to the Biblical version, the woman does not spring from the rib of a man, but instead it appears that the male brain, and male physiology in general, are variations of the female master plan. Early in utero, differences in the amount of male hormone testosterone give rise to changes in both the male and female brain. In some mammals, the ensuing dimorphism (from the Greek *dimorphos*, to have two forms) is rather marked, but this is not the case with humans.

In the human brain, it is difficult to detect gross structural changes related to gender outside of the hypothalamus and perhaps the corpus callosum. The male and the female are to be found on a continuum where differences in the human brain are found only between the averages of the genders. It is not yet known how gender differences in the brain compare with differences between random individuals of either gender. This makes it difficult to determine how an individual brain compares to the average, and to determine the gender of an unlabelled brain. There is not necessarily a relationship between a person's sex, brain, and secondary sexual characteristics. For example, that means that a person can have a body that appears male in the extreme, but a brain that is closer to the female extreme.

Gender differences in brain processing continue to fascinate the public, and stereotypes abound, including that women are comparably poorer at navigation, and men, at verbalizing their emotions. There may well be a scientific basis to these presumed differences, but they are unlikely to be linked to genetic differences. Instead, if they are real, they are probably a product of learning and linked to the way gender shapes expectations and functioning during a person's upbringing. However, such gender differences are small compared with the natural human variation across sex, and it remains difficult to detect them with brain imaging.

SEX ON THE BRAIN

Humans are driven by desires in similar ways as other animals are. Sex is very clear example of this. In animals such as elephants, sex has a reproductive purpose, and even if sex appears to carry its own reward, it is rarely used recreationally in normal members of most animal species.

However, in some primate species such as bonobos, it is clear that recreational sex serves as a very strong agent for social cohesion. The joy of sex is clearly present in these intelligent apes. In many other animals, there are marked differences between the male and female physiology and thus also in the brain. Such dimorphisms are more difficult to find in the human brain, and while they may exist, it is perhaps worth asking to what extent they have significant behavioral consequences. At this time, we do not yet know enough about such differences to warrant more than speculations that claim that the inherent structure of the brain makes men or women do this or that and is therefore impossible to change. This could easily become an excuse for the status quo of current gender relations.

With regards to the brain mechanisms of sexual behavior, it is clear that sex draws upon the same brain regions that are used in other drives, such as food and drugs. Sex is also subject to the same mechanisms of selective satiation, which means that it may be advantageous to vary one's behavior and that too much of a good thing really can be too much. As in so many other areas, variety is the spice of life. But first and foremost, we need more data to be able to be more specific with regard to the sexual brain.

It is too early to say much about where romantic love may be represented in the human brain. Of course there are sub-aspects of love such as social attachment and maternal love that are meaningful to study. But we are far from understanding the brain correlates of romantic love. It is difficult to switch romantic love on and off continuously, which is what would be required to study love with brain scanning. Some studies have claimed to have investigated romantic love by comparing the activity related to the faces of loved ones compared to that of other faces. Alas, such comparisons based on subtractions of brain activity may in fact miss the very thing studied, because being in love is a pervasive ongoing state that is not switched off when we see the face of someone we do not love.

However, some inferences can be drawn about the neural correlates of love from the other findings presented in this book. It would seem likely that love would draw upon the same brain regions and neurotransmitters as those implicated in the other desires and pleasures of the emotional brain. This means that regions of the orbitofrontal and cingulate cortices are likely to be important for love, just as they are important for food, sex, and drugs.

● ● ● HAPPINESS LESSON

Sex is for more than reproduction, and there are examples of this in nature beyond just human behavior. Given the great diversity of sex in the world, "unnatural acts" usually aren't unnatural at all (except, perhaps, chastity).

FURTHER READING

Sexual behavior is found in many animals and rarely more human-like than in bonobos, as described in, de Waal, F. B. M. & Lanting, F. (1997). *Bonobo: The Forgotten Ape.* London: University of California Press, Berkeley.

But of course bonobos are not humans, and few researchers have matched the ability of Kinsey to describe the mechanical aspects of human desire: Kinsey, A. C. (1953). *Sexual Behavior in the Human Female.* (Institute for Sex Research), Philadelphia; London: Saunders. Kinsey, A. C., Pomeroy, W. B. & Martin, C. E. (1948). *Sexual Behavior in the Human Male.* London, Philadelphia: W. Saunders.

These books revolutionized our knowledge of that goes on behind the blinds and have since been extended in books such as: Masters, W. & Johnson, V. (1966). *Human Sexual Response.* Boston: Little & Brown.

11

FUTURE CONSIDERATIONS

Where Do We Go From Here?

> As I walk through this wicked world
> Searching for light in the darkness of insanity.
> I ask myself, Is all hope lost?
> Is there only pain, and hatred, and misery?
> And each time I feel like this inside, there's one thing
> I wanna know:
> What's so funny 'bout peace love and understanding?
>
> Nick Lowe (1949–)

THE HAPPINESS OF DAILY LIFE

As shown in this book, the pleasure center of the brain is not a center that one can visit to extract more pleasure. Rather it is a complex entity consisting of a republic of connected brain regions, whose activity changes dynamically over time and is seldom fully available for conscious introspection. Neuroscience can help to uncover this constant maelstrom of brain activity. Our journey to the pleasure center is therefore not foremost an exploration of consciousness as such but perhaps rather an exploration of the nonconscious brain processes which lead to choices and actions—and even pleasure.

Pleasure, desire, and happiness coexist in consciousness. We can ask people how they are consciously experiencing their pleasure and contentment at any given time. But their answers are not necessarily informative, since we are not particularly skilled at decoding our subjective states and nonconscious brain activity. There can be huge differences between how we say we should feel and how we do feel.

But what is it that we say that we like? In order to answer this question, Daniel Kahneman and colleagues had almost a 1000 American women reconstruct their working day and rate each activity. Perhaps not surprisingly the women found that having sex was the best part of their day. But this lasted, on average, only 0.2 hours and only 11% of the women had this pleasure on that particular day.

Socialising with friends was reported by the majority of the women and was the second most pleasurable activity during the day. Eating and relaxing was also very pleasurable for the women. So the women were like most people who will self-report that they get enjoyment out of the sensory, sexual, and social pleasures.

They also reported that commuting and working were what they disliked most during their day. Perhaps surprisingly they also reported that being with their children was less rewarding than watching television or shopping. (Some mothers stated that while, in general, they really enjoy being with their kids, on that particular day the kids were being horrible.) Interestingly, the women also found the time with friends and relatives more rewarding than time with their partner or their children.

This study of hedonic processing also confirmed what many other studies have found previously. The increase in wealth over the last 50 years in the developed countries has had little or no influence on quality of life and happiness. This has been called the paradox of the *hedonic treadmill.* Our quality of life may change temporarily with changes in fortunes such as winning the lottery or divorce, but with time it will eventually come back to the same level.

Many hypotheses have been put forward to account for this paradox. One of the most popular is our inability to focus. Our attention is often framed by our current circumstances and even by the way the questions are posed. In one study, some students were asked first about how happy they were with life in general and then how many dates they had been on this month. When the questions were posed in this order, there was no significant correlation between the answers as might otherwise have been expected. If the questions were posed the other way round, there was, however, a very high correlation.

Money Can't Buy Love

Many people tend to think that having a high income must be related to a better quality of life, but research has shown this to be mostly illusionary. People with high incomes (>$100,000) usually report being relatively content but seldom report feeling more content in day-to-day experiences, are far more tense, and use less time on leisure activities than those with lower incomes.

Yet, many people are strongly motivated to increase their income and will accept doing things that are clearly not pleasurable—such as longer commutes and working hours—in order to achieve this goal.

This is likely to stem from our inability to correctly predict both our own and other pleasure states. In another study on hardworking American women, Kahneman and colleagues asked them to characterize the events of their day in four mood categories ranging from really poor to very good. They were also asked to predict the mood states of women in other circumstances such as different income (low, high), marital status (alone or married), and with or without health insurance.

Given that the researchers had chosen women from all of these categories, they were able to compare how these women self-reported their mood and how other women thought they would report their mood.

Not surprisingly there were some differences in negative mood states between the different groups of women, with for example, less negative mood in the high-income group than in the low-income group. But the most striking and significant differences were between the predicted and the actual scores for the different groups, where for example, most women predicted that the low-income group would be in a bad mood two-thirds of the time, when in fact they were only in a bad mood a third of the time. Generally there were around 25 to 40% points between the predictions and the actual self-reports.

The women were thus prone to exaggeration and seemingly unable to predict how other women would feel when their circumstances differed from their own. This may in part be explainable by a lack of focus and attention to the relevant factors. We become used to our circumstances and with time we no longer view them as relevant background when making reports on our quality of life. This is why winning the lottery or divorcing mostly have only transient effects on our lives. While we happily predict that they would change our lives forever, in reality this almost never happens.

Our subjective pleasures are more likely to come from events in our daily lives. Over the long term we get far more pleasure out of being with friends and enjoying good food, music, and sex than we do from winning the lottery.

HEDONIC TIME TRAVEL

The brain's reward and pleasure systems help not only us but also other animals survive and reproduce. One of the most important goals of any animal is to become sufficiently skilled at predicting the influence of future events on their level of pleasure and reward. Even if we have not seen or experienced a fire, we learn to heed the sound of fire alarm, just in case.

Once we have learned the pleasure of chocolate, even briefest of glimpses of chocolate wrapping can awaken our desire. In the same way, even the slightest sniff of fire may be enough for us to try to escape. Pleasure and pain are in many ways the guiding stars of our journey through life.

Some researchers have proposed that humans are much better than other animals at predicting future events, since only we have the ability to imagine hypothetical situations we have never experienced before. We can even imagine how situations may make us feel and which pleasures or pains await us.

Unfortunately, despite the rumours of our advanced mental abilities, we are in fact not very good at predicting our hedonic experience of imaginary future events. Our expectations and dreams of clandestine love affairs with for example, teachers or handymen do apparently seldom compare favourably with the actual experience. Very few of us would expect to enjoy eating a combination of liquorice and asparagus, and yet this is what many guests will report after having visiting restaurants serving molecular gastronomy.

Our ability to predict the future is in many ways related to our ability to empathize, to put ourselves in someone else's shoes. On the basis of our emotional experiences our brain can pretend "as if" we were other people or experiencing future events right now. It is far better to be able to imagine meeting a tiger and working out how to get away in advance, rather than to have to make this calculation on the spot.

This mental simulation is thus dependent on our powers of imagination. We can try to fool the brain by inventing sensory impressions, but this fantasy will often lack the power of the actual sensory stimuli. This is why our subjective experience of meeting an imaginary tiger is often a poor substitute for meeting a real tiger. Even if our mental simulations and predictions allow us to make hedonic time travel to the future, these experiences are seldom comparable to our actual experiences.

Just as the working women were poor at predicting the mood states of other women unlike themselves, we have only a fleeting insight into our future pleasures. This most likely stems from our lack of ability to focus on or even recognize that which gives us real pleasure.

We may think that winning the lottery or becoming CEO at a prestigious company will help our quality of life. This is not always the case, and a friend of mine who has achieved the latter reported that she gets more satisfaction from simple pleasures such as being able to afford a house that allows her to walk to work, rather than having a long commute.

In Pursuit of Happiness and Love

Simple pleasures usually work best for our contentment and quality of life. We are beginning to understand how a very large role for this quality of life is played by the early attachment process between parents and children.

This is perhaps best illustrated through postnatal depression, which is common, occurring in approximately 13% of mothers and 3% of fathers after birth and often within 6 weeks. Postnatal depression has been associated with a range of adverse child outcomes including behavioral and emotional disturbances and attachment, and there is also some evidence for poorer cognitive outcomes. There is increasing evidence that certain features of the behavior of depressed mothers are associated with adverse outcome, in particular their lack of responsiveness to the infant, the reduced ability to perceive their infant's signals, and less mimetic behavior with a resultant lack of contingency between the infant's actions and the mother's responses. Furthermore, it has been shown experimentally that infants respond adversely with distress, crying, increased arousal, and then avoidance to an unresponsive maternal face.

In order to improve the pleasures of the general population, it is therefore paramount that we get better at identifying the early signs of postnatal depression and find better ways of treating it, in order to improve the emotional balance.

But parental love is not the only love that matters. Romantic love clearly plays a very significant role in our lives. As we saw earlier, many of the stimuli that lead to this state are not necessarily consciously experienced. We feel the butterflies in our stomach and interpret this as love—but it might also be something we ate.

One of my close friends was fully aware of the research on the nonconscious influences on emotion and pleasure. He was hopelessly in love with another student but unfortunately she had not revealed any strong feelings on her part. They were due to go to a conference in a hotel near a beach. He therefore put together a cunning plan of getting the two of them on one of those speedboats shaped like bananas. He was hoping that the excitement would make her realize her true feelings for him.

She reluctantly came along for the ride. Afterwards she was shaken and excited in equal measures, but sadly she was unable to stop telling him how handsome she found the driver of the speedboat.

Concluding Remarks About Happiness

Depression, mania, schizophrenia, and other mental illnesses have caused so much suffering to so many people that we need all the help we can get. Even if there is darkness in the depth of the malignant emotions, and suicide seems like the only way out, it is important to get correct and timely information about how to recover. There is always hope—even if it may at times seem like only a glimmer. At the end of the day, it is other people who make it worth staying on and who can help us back to the pleasure and happiness of life.

But what is the relationship between desire, pleasure, and happiness? Might happiness be best described as pleasure without desire, a state of contentment and indifference? Such a state is perhaps akin to the kind of bliss that Buddhists seek through meditation.

If so, it is possible that neuroscientists may one day find ways to help induce this state. Then we might have a chance of a true utilitarian society in which overall happiness can be maximized, as the eighteenth century philosopher Jeremy Bentham proposed. The question of whether such a society would be desirable and even pleasurable remains to be answered.

Meanwhile it is worth remembering that we are all, to some extent, able to control our measure of pleasure and desire. We can choose to spend our time in activities that are related to the *fluid absorption* mentioned earlier. This is a state of self-forgetfulness that is present in activities that afford us deep pleasure without external reward.

Some people experience fluid absorption when skiing, climbing, or swimming. Others may also experience this deep, intense feeling when playing with their children or socializing with good friends or when writing, or playing football. It is a state of happiness that is always potentially present in our lives. It is not about orgasmic pleasure but rather about exploring the potential for pleasure in the now, without wanting to be elsewhere. We are far from understanding the functional neuroanatomy of this deep state, but this is of course one of the main goals for the affective neuroscience of pleasure.

● STILL TO COME

This book argues that the study of pleasure could be the central tool in understanding human nature, so it should be reintegrated into the cognitive brain sciences. Using stimuli such as food, sex, and drugs can give us precise information about the neural correlates of pleasure and aversion. Our subjective experience is perhaps *the* defining characteristic of consciousness. As we have seen, several brain regions are possible candidates for mediating this experience. The orbitofrontal cortex, anterior cingulate cortex, insular cortex, ventral pallidum, and ventral striatum have been clearly implicated in the hedonic networks that contribute to shaping our behavior and our subjective experience.

The interplay between brain, body, and environment is complex. The brain integrates sensory impressions of the environment with body states and needs, to allow for the best possible decisions and behavior. This integration includes the active processes of desire, pleasure, and emotion to take past experience and expectation into account to ultimately bring about at least two kinds of change: *external change* in the form of muscle movements, whether they be large-scale limb movements or speech (as already pointed out by the English neurophysiologist Charles Sherrington), and *internal change* to our bodily organs such as that seen in fight-or-flight behavior, which can cause changes in heart rhythm, and production of sweat and gastric acids.

Both kinds of changes become part of the complex feedback systems that in turn cause changes in the functional organization of the brain in the form of learning, memories, and thoughts, which help us to adapt future behavior. We are able to report on some aspects of these changes, but such rationalizations are often post-hoc. Learning more about these changes through careful application of brain-monitoring techniques discussed throughout the preceding chapters will greatly advance our understanding of human nature and consciousness.

BROADENING OUR OUTLOOK

Humans are constantly searching for meaning, often as connections between objects and sensory qualities from the outside world. Our senses are limited by our genes, but over time, culture has acquired a life of its own with the invention of metaphors and allocation of new meaning. An understanding of human nature can come only through an understanding of the interplay between genes and culture. It is difficult to see how this can come about separately in traditional disciplines such as the sciences or the humanities. It is perhaps better treated as a whole with recognition of our evolutionary history.

This means that the complex systems seen in the social sciences might gain from using tools from other disciplines such as neuroscience, biology, psychology, and physics. By the same token, these scientific disciplines could equally gain from the tools of the social sciences. In fact, the really difficult science may be the complex systems of the social sciences rather than those seen in the so-called hard sciences.

According to quite a few studies, humans are foremost interested in the fundamentals of life: sex, family, work, security, personal expression, entertainment, and spirituality. Many people see the sciences as peripheral to these goals, while the humanities and social sciences are much more intimately related.

Is this really true? The scientific instinct is, as art also is, a universal attribute of humanity, and scientific knowledge is a vital part of the repertoire of our species. The beginning of the twenty first century has seen an exponential increase in the access to factual knowledge in our privileged Western cultures. This has been primarily linked to the rise in scientific technologies. We may be drowning in information, but we are still thirsting for wisdom. It will be crucial to synthesize knowledge from many fields.

This knowledge can then be applied to the problems of the world on the most basic levels. As discussed earlier, we socially mirror ourselves in other people. We use much of our time second-guessing their intentions, pleasures, desires, and motives. This is a different form than that which is claimed by professional mind readers. Mind reading in social relations is the innate ability of humans to represent and understand the behavior of others. We translate the behavior of other individuals into an understanding of sensations, expectations, and goals. Though on a basic level we have managed to do this well enough to perpetuate our species, misunderstandings continue to produce clashes, sometimes violent, between individuals, between groups, and between countries. Better understanding of basic motivations and urges will improve our judgment and decision-making and help us avoid some, although not all, conflicts.

TO INFINITY AND BEYOND?

The challenges we face are ever increasing and have been since we began to pursue technological progress about 10,000 years ago. Advanced technology has become the ultimate human prosthesis and, with the continuing increase in population growth, an ever-greater pressure on resources causes changes in the climate. We will have to learn to control our impact on the environment before it is too late.

Given our technological progress, we are not only at the threshold of improving our understanding of human nature, but possibly also of changing human genetic nature. This could be the beginning of a unique epoch in human history, which will require wisdom to manage.

It should stimulate action that, even in the most optimistic analyses, the Earth can support only around 16 billion vegetarians (which would not leave much biodiversity). Thus the question of how to best use the Earth's resources becomes ever more pressing. At a time when we are getting better at measuring the activity of the living brain to improve our understanding of ourselves, we are undermining our very survival as a species.

Radical new solutions seem needed. Some have been offered by those carefree prophets of prosperity who, driven by an unlimited enthusiasm for new technologies, carry the mantle of the science-fiction writers of the 1950s. Why limit ourselves to solving our current environmental and resource problems? Why not opt for an exit strategy whereby humanity populates other planets, as the first humans probably left Africa to occupy the rest of the Earth? It may be hard to see how we can find the resources to colonize other planets, but Mars has always beckoned. Placed in environments fundamentally different from Earth, the instincts our species has honed for quick response to many situations may often no longer fit the circumstances. In these cases, a thorough knowledge of why we react the ways we do will be required if we are to rechannel our responses to more appropriate actions.

But the most radical solution can take place right here on Earth.

A MATTER OF PERSPECTIVE

Many of the problems facing the world arise from, or are exacerbated by, short-term thinking based on the human desire for rewards that will arrive immediately or in the near future. Perhaps we need a project that can help to slow the pace. The now and the future is a product of the past. As the

Polish poet Wislawa Szymborska wrote "when I pronounce the word Future, the first syllable already belongs to the past." But how long is *the now*? For most of us *the now* is this week haunted by the ghost of last week, or perhaps rather *the now* where we act and still think ourselves able to assess its consequences. In other words, we appear to be limited in our hedonic projections.

But if we continue to rush from moment to moment, how are we ever going to be able to get the energy to represent and project the distant future? What if we decided to change *the now* to include a 100 years in each direction, which would include the previous and coming generations? Maybe this would give us some more space and a better overview.

In fact, why not include even larger periods of time into *the now*? After all, our current civilization is not older than around 10,000 years. Seen in this perspective, everything looks rather different.

Of course it is not possible to change our perception of *the now*, but it might be useful to search for that which might be called *the long now*. That might be similar to the perspectives of Zen Buddhists, who are taught to observe infinite gratitude for the past, infinite service to the present, and infinite responsibility for the future.

The American physicist Freeman Dyson has proposed that time exists on six different scales. Years are on the scale of individuals, decades belong to families, centuries to groups or nations, millennia to cultures, tens of millennia to species, and eternity to all life. Every person is governed by all of these scales. When people are said to be complex, it is because our demands come from all of these scales, which are themselves complex and often directly conflicting.

Another model of time comes from Stewart Brand, who has proposed a spiral, layered classification of time changes, thus civilizations. The layers have a built-in fast speed in which the outer layers are always faster and more innovative than the stabilizing inner layers. Each of these layers counteracts and influences the other layers. Outermost is fashion, followed by commerce overlying infrastructure. Underneath this layer is one government overlying culture, which supports the innermost layer, Nature.

IN THE LONG RUN

The rapidly changing layers of culture can be likened to a dog being kept on a leash by a human nature that has not changed in the time we have been *Homo Sapiens sapiens*, the wise primate. So we may experiment with alternative ways of living and smart technological gadgets, but in the long run, what really matters for the survival of the species is to produce new offspring and make sure they are adequately fed.

Partly as a result of our technological advances, we are overpopulated, which is increasing pressure on the climate. It is too early to predict whether we will be able to solve this problem with advanced technology—or whether this problem may solve itself. But it is increasingly clear that we need wise decisions (Figure 11.1).

We will need patience and control of our more destructive desires and pleasures if we are to successfully face tomorrow's hard challenges, possibly including continued

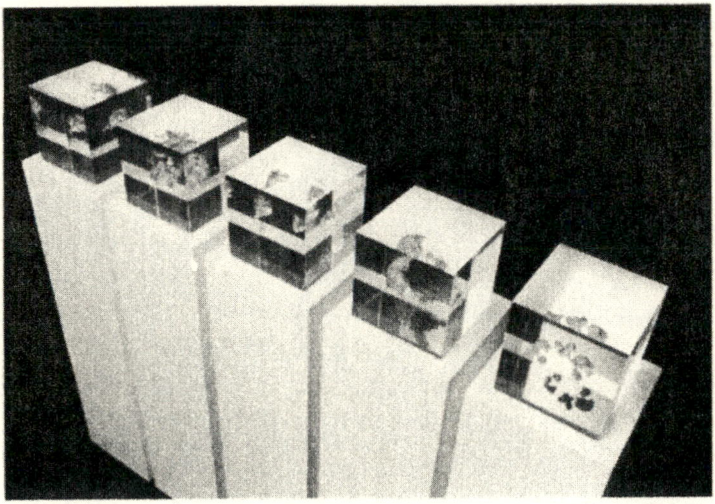

Figure 11.1 Brain portraits. The collaboration with artist Annie Cattrell resulted in five sculptures of the brain activity related to the five senses. The sculptures were made using the rapid prototyping technique and was purchased by the Wellcome Trust for their permanent collection. They can be thought of as a radical reinterpretation of the art of portraiture.

overpopulation, abrupt climate change, and even other beings with artificial consciousness. Human nature and the tragic miracle of consciousness will undoubtedly be tested to the fullest. We will need large amounts of patience, but at the same time it may be worth remembering that the more things change, the more they remain the same.

At the Society for Neuroscience meeting mentioned in Chapter 8, the Dalai Lama reminded the scientific audience of the "fundamental values of compassion and affection" that are "important to the development of body and brain." It would seem prudent for future research on happiness, pleasure, and desire not to ignore this compassionate plea for human dignity while tinkering with the very core of what makes us human.

Linking Pleasure and Happiness

Happiness is both very difficult to define and to induce with any regularity. In addition, it is usually only after the fact that we know whether we were happy or not. The scientific study of happiness is therefore still in its infancy. Some questionnaire studies have investigated well-being but the answers are highly dependent on how the questions are posed. Still, some preliminary results of these studies suggest that material wealth above a certain minimum has limited influence on well-being but that the fundamental sensory, sexual, and social pleasures are very important. In particular, the social interactions appear to be very important for our happiness.

Happiness is perhaps best described as liking without wanting as a stable state of contentment and can be found in deep states such as fluid absorption. Happiness is seldom present when pleasure is missing, anhedonia, which is a common feature of mental illness. A better understanding of the neurobiology of pleasure can therefore help to optimize the amount of pleasure in the general population and perhaps even add a bit of happiness.

NOTES

1 The Challenge

5 **Pleasure is defined and described in great detail** in our review article Berridge, K. C. & Kringelbach, M. L. (2008) Affective neuroscience of pleasure: Reward in humans and animals. *Psychopharmacology* 199, 457–480. doi:10.1007/s00213-008-1099-6. In addition, we have gathered **the views of the world experts on pleasure** in our forthcoming edited book: Kringelbach, M. L. & Berridge, K. C. (2008) *Pleasures of the Brain*. New York, NY: Oxford University Press.

5 The **relation of pleasure to emotion** is described in Frijda, N. E. (2006). *The Laws of Emotion*. New York: Lawrence Erlbaum Associates.

6 An excellent overview to Berridge's **research on wanting and liking** can be found in Berridge, K. C. (1996). Food reward: Brain substrates of wanting and liking. *Neuroscience and Biobehavioral Reviews*. 20, 1–25.

7 **Desire** is described in great detail in the book Schroeder, T. (2004). *Three Faces of Desire*. Oxford: Oxford University Press.

2 Decisions

13 A good collection of articles on **chimpanzee cultures** are collected in the book Wrangham, R. W., McGrew, W. C.,

de Waal, F. B. M. & Heltne, P. (1994). *Chimpanzee Cultures.* Cambridge, MA: Harvard University Press.

13 **Mirror neurons** were first described in Rizzolatti, G., Camarda, R., Fogassi, L., Gentilucci, M., Luppino, G. & Matelli, M. (1988). Functional organization of inferior area 6 in the macaque monkey. Area F5 and the control of distal movements. *Experimental Brain Research.* 71, 491–507.

13 Gallup's research on **self-recognition** started with the following paper: Gallup, G. G. (1970) Chimpanzees: Self-recognition. *Science.* 167, 86–7.

16 Our study on the **cuteness of infant faces** can be found in Kringelbach, M. L., Lehtonen, A., Squire, S., Harvey, A., Craske, M. G., Holliday, I. E., Green, A. L., Aziz, T. Z., Hansen, P. C., Cornelissen, P. L. & Stein, A. (2007b). Infant faces evoke a highly specific and rapid neural response in adults. PLoS ONE, 3(2): e1664. doi:10.1371/journal.pone.0001664.

18 More information on the **IQ of adopted children** can be found in Duyme, M., Dumaret, A. C. & Tomkiewicz, S. (1999). How can we boost IQs of "dull children?": A late adoption study. *Proceedings of The National Academy of Sciences of The United States of America.* 96, 8790–4.

20 The classic description of the **action potential of neurons** is described in the article Hodgkin, A. L. & Huxley, A. F. (1952). A quantitative description of membrane current and its application to conduction and excitation in nerve. *Journal Of Physiology (London).* 117, 500–44.

20 The **details of cortical neurons** can be found in the book Braitenberg, V. & Schüz, A. (1998) *Cortex: Statistics and Geometry of Neuronal Connectivity,* 2nd ed, *Anatomy of the Cortex: Statistics and Geometry* 1991, New York, NY: Springer, Berlin Heidelberg.

21 **Hebb's law** is described in the book Hebb, D. O. (1949). *Organization of Behaviour: A Neuropsychological Theory. Stimulus and Response—and What Occurs in the Brain in the Interval Between Them.* New York, NY: Wiley.

21 **Neural networks in the brain** are described for the layman in the book Cotterill, R. M. J. (1998). *Enchanted Looms.*

Conscious Networks in Brains and Computers. Cambridge: Cambridge University Press.

22 **Lesions of the orbitofrontal cortex in monkeys** were described in the classic paper Iversen, S. D. & Mishkin, M. (1970). Perseverative interference in monkeys following selective lesions of the inferior prefrontal convexity. *Experimental Brain Research.* 11, 376–86.

23 The **Iowa gambling task** was first described in Bechara, A., Damasio, A. R., Damasio, H. & Anderson, S. W. (1994). Insensitivity to future consequences following damage to human prefrontal cortex. *Cognition.* 50, 7–15.

23 Our **probabilistic reversal task** is described in O'Doherty, J., Kringelbach, M. L., Rolls, E. T., Hornak, J. & Andrews, C. (2001). Abstract reward and punishment representations in the human orbitofrontal cortex. *Nature Neuroscience.* 4, 95–102.

24 Our paper on **social decisions based on facial expressions** Kringelbach, M. L. & Rolls, E. T. (2003). Neural correlates of rapid context-dependent reversal learning in a simple model of human social interaction. *Neuroimage.* 20, 1371–83.

25 The **illusion of conscious free will** is eloquently explained in Wegner, D. M. (2002). *The Illusion of Conscious Will.* Cambridge, MA: MIT Press.

25 **Irrationality** is applauded in a fine, small book Sutherland, S. (1992). *Irrationality. The enemy within.* London: Constable and Co.

26 **The readiness potential** was first described in the paper Kornhuber,H.H.&Deecke,L.(1965).Hirnpotentialänderungen bei willkürbewegungen und passiven bewegungen des menschen: Bereitschaftspotential und reafferente potentiale. *Pflûgers Arch: European Journal of Physiology.* 284, 1–17.

26 **Libet's ideas on free will** can be found in the following paper among other places: Libet, B., Gleason, C. A., Wright, E. W. & Pearl, D. K. (1983). Time of conscious intention to act in relation to onset of cerebral activity (readinesspotential). The unconscious initiation of a freely voluntary act. *Brain.* 106, 623–42.

28 **Unconscious liking** was found in the experiment described in Winkielman, P., Berridge, K. C. & Wilbarger, J. L. (2005). Unconscious affective reactions to masked happy versus angry faces influence consumption behavior and judgments of value. *Personality and Social Psychology Bulletin.* 31, 121–35.

3 Consciousness

30 John Steinbeck is mostly known for *Grapes of Wrath*, but he also wrote presciently **about consciousness**: Steinbeck, J. & Ricketts, E. F. (1941). *The Log from the Sea of Cortez.* London: Penguin.

32 **REM sleep in humans** was first described in the article Aserinsky, E. & Kleitman, N. (1953). Regularly occurring periods of eye motility and concomitant phenomena during sleep. *Science.* 118, 273–4.

37 A good description of the history and dilemmas of **evolutionary psychology** can be found in the book Laland, K. N. & Brown, G. (2002). *Sense and Nonsense: Evolutionary Perspectives on Human Behaviour.* New York, NY: Oxford University Press.

38 More about **Dawkins' evolutionary ideas** in his classic book Dawkins, R. (1976). *The Selfish Gene.* Oxford: Oxford University Press. His latest book is written with **fundamentalist fervor**: Dawkins, R. (2006) *The God Delusion.* London: Bantam Books.

41 Walter Burkert gave the **Gifford-lectures on religion**, which was since made into an excellent book Burkert, W. (1996). *The Creation of the Sacred. Tracks of Biology in Early Religions.* Cambridge, MA: Harvard University Press.

42 **Movement** as a point of departure: "To move things is all mankind can do, and for such the sole executant is muscle, whether in whispering a syllable or in felling a forest," Charles Sherrington, 1924 *Linacre Lectures*—as cited on page 59 in the book: Eccles, J. C. & Gibson, W. C.

(1979). *Sherrington. His Life and Thought.* New York, NY: Springer. In addition, many interesting observations about **the human brain** can be found in the book: Sherrington, C. S. (1951). *Man on His Nature.* Cambridge: Cambridge University Press.

4 Emotions

47 **High anxiety** can be reinterpreted as attraction: Dutton, D. G. & Aron, A. P. (1974). Some evidence for heightened sexual attraction under conditions of high anxiety. *Journal of Personality and Social Psychology.* 30, 510–17.

48 More on **Darwin and emotions** can be found in the classic Darwin, C. (1872). *The Expression of the Emotions in Man and Animals.* Chicago: University of Chicago Press.

49 The **James–Lange's theory** on emotional experience can be found in the books James, W. (1890). *The Principles of Psychology.* New York: Henry Holt. Lange, C. G. (1887). *Über Gemüstbewegungen. (Dansk org. Om Sindsbevægelser),* Leipzig.

49 **Cannon's critique of James-Lange's theory** can be found in the paper Cannon, W. B. (1927). The James-Lange theory of emotion. *American Journal of Psychology.* 39, 106–24.

49 Nauta's **interoceptive marker** theory was described in Nauta, W. J. (1971). The problem of the frontal lobe: A reinterpretation. *Journal of Psychiatric Research.* 8, 167–87. Damasio's **somatic marker theory** was described in the book: Damasio, A. R. (1994). *Descartes' Error.* New York, NY: Putnam.

50 The brain pathways for **interoception** are described in Craig, A. D. (2002). Opinion: How do you feel? Interoception: The sense of the physiological condition of the body. *Nature Reviews Neuroscience.* 3, 655–66.

51 **Pavlov's life** is described in the book Gray, J. A. (1979). *Ivan Pavlov.* New York, NY: Viking Press.

51 Thorndike laid the **foundation for behaviorism** in the book Thorndike, E. L. (1911). *Animal Intelligence: Experimental Studies*. New York, NY: Macmillan.

52 **Behaviorism** found its high priest and gospel in Skinner, B. F. (1938). *The Behavior of Organisms: An Experimental Analysis*. New York: Appleton-Century.

52 The potentially **detrimental effects of reward** are documented in Lepper, M. R., Greene, D. & Nisbett, R. E. (1973). Undermining children's intrinsic interest with extrinsic reward: A test of the overjustification hypothesis. *Journal of Personality and Social Psychology*. 28, 129–37.

54 A very readable introduction to the **importance of the amygdala for emotions** can be found in the book LeDoux, J. E. (1996). *The Emotional Brain*. New York, NY: Simon and Schuster.

54 A good review article on the **anatomy of the amygdala**: Swanson, L. W. & Petrovich, G. D. (1998). What is the amygdala? *Trends in Neurosciences*. 21, 323–31.

55 Olds and Milner's research on **electrical self-stimulation in the rat** was first described in Olds, J. & Milner, P. (1954). Positive reinforcement produced by electrical stimulation of the septal area and other regions of rat brain. *Journal of Comparative and Physiological Psychology*. 47, 419–27.

56 An example of Robert Heath's research on **self-stimulation in humans** can be found in Heath, R. G. (1963). Electrical self-stimulation of the brain in man. *American Journal of Psychiatry*. 120, 571–7.

56 The **hedonic hot spots in the brain** are described in Peciña, S. & Berridge, K. C. (2005). Hedonic hot spot in nucleus accumbens shell: Where do mu-opioids cause increased hedonic impact of sweetness? *Journal of Neuroscience*. 25, 11777–86.

57 Early **drive theories of motivation** include the following: Hull, C. L. (1951). *Essentials of behavior*. New Haven, CT: Yale University Press. Bindra, D. (1978). How adaptive behavior is produced: A perceptual-motivational alternative to response-reinforcement. *Behavioral and Brain Sciences*. 1, 41–91.

57 The phenomenon of **allisthesia** is described in the classic paper Cabanac, M. (1971). Physiological role of pleasure. *Science.* 173, 1103–7.

57 The **dissociation of wanting and liking** is eloquently described in Berridge, K. C. (1996). Food reward: brain substrates of wanting and liking. *Neuroscience and Biobehavioral Reviews.* **20**, 1–25.

58 Ekman's pioneering research on **facial expressions** is described in Ekman, P. & Friesen, W.-V. (1971) Constants across cultures in the face and emotion. *Journal of Personality and Social Psychology* 17(2), 124–129. Ekman, P. (1982) *Emotion in the Human Face.* Cambridge University Press, Cambridge.

59 The main source for our limited information **on Phineas Gage** comes from two articles: Harlow, J. M. (1848). Passage of an iron rod through the head. *Boston Medical and Surgical Journal.* 39, 389–93. Harlow, J. (1868). Recovery after severe injury to the head. *Massachusetts Medical Society Publications.* 2, 327–47. This has not stopped a litany of **inflated and untrue stories** about Phineas Gage, as uncovered in the book: Macmillan, M. (2000). *An Odd Kind of Fame: Stories of Phineas Gage.* Cambridge, MA: MIT Press.

59 The concept of **the limbic system** was initiated by Paul Broca in the paper, Broca, P. (1878). Anatomie comparée des circonvolutions cérébrales: Le grand lobe limbique et le scissure limbique dans la série des mammifères. *Rev d'Anthrop Par.* 3.s, 385–498. This idea was then taken over by **James Papez** in his influential emotion paper Papez, J. W. (1927). A proposed mechanism for emotion. *Archives of Neurology and Psychiatry.* 38, 725–43. The idea, however, was taken to **its logical extreme** by Paul MacLean: MacLean, P. (1949). Psychosomatic disease and the "visceral brain": Recent developments bearing on the Papez theory of emotion. *Psychosomatic Medicine.* 11, 338–53. MacLean, P. (1990) *The Triune Brain in Evolution.* New York, NY: Plenum Press.

60 The **brain mechanisms for selective satiety** in the brain are described in Kringelbach, M. L., O'Doherty, J., Rolls, E. T. & Andrews, C. (2003). Activation of the human orbitofrontal cortex to a liquid food stimulus is correlated with its subjective pleasantness. *Cerebral Cortex.* 13, 1064–71.

62 The **combination of DBS and MEG** can be found in Kringelbach, M. L., Jenkinson, N., Green, A. L., Owen, S. L. F., Hansen, P. C., Cornelissen, P. L., Holliday, I. E., Stein, J. & Aziz, T. Z. (2007). Deep brain stimulation for chronic pain investigated with magnetoencephalography. *Neuroreport.* 8(3), 223–8.

63 Henrik **Nordbrandt's childhood** is described in his excellent memoir Nordbrandt, H. (2002). *Døden fra Lübeck.* Gyldendal, Copenhagen.

64 **Harry Harlow's life** is well captured in the book Blum, D. (2002). *Love at Goon Park: Harry Harlow and the Science of Affection.* New York, NY: Perseus Publishing.

65 Harry **Harlow's experiments** can, for example, be found, in the article Harlow, H. F. (1958). The nature of love. *The American Psychologist.* 13, 673–85.

68 Our initial research using **brain scanning of gambling**: O'Doherty, J., Kringelbach, M. L., Rolls, E. T., Hornak, J. & Andrews, C. (2001). Abstract reward and punishment representations in the human orbitofrontal cortex. *Nature Neuroscience.* 4, 95–102.

5 Sensation

75 Description of the **selective devaluation of the subjective sensory experience** from a set-point such as hunger can be found in Cabanac, M. (1971). Physiological role of pleasure. *Science.* 173, 1103–7. Rolls, B. J., Rolls, E. T., Rowe, E. A. & Sweeney, K. (1981) Sensory specific satiety in man. *Physiology and Behavior.* 27, 137–42.

77 Our research group has investigated the cortical representation of **the fifth taste, umami,** in the human brain: De Araujo, I. E. T., Kringelbach, M. L., Rolls, E. T. & Hobden, P. (2003). The representation of umami taste in the human brain. *Journal of Neurophysiology.* 90, 313–9.

79 Our research group found **taste-related information in dorsolateral prefrontal cortex**: Kringelbach, M. L., de Araujo, I. E. T. & Rolls, E. T. (2004). Taste-related activity in the human dorsolateral prefrontal cortex. *Neuroimage.* 21, 781–8.

83 The discussion on **pheromones in the human brain** can be found in the articles Monti-Bloch, L., Jennings-White, C. & Berliner, D. L. (1998). The human vomeronasal system. A review. *Annals of the New York Academy of Sciences.* 855, 373–89. Stern, K. & McClintock, M. K. (1998) Regulation of ovulation by human pheromones. *Nature.* 392, 177–9.

83 **Women's T-shirt preference** is described in Wedekind, C., Seebeck, T., Bettens, F. & Paepke, A. J. (1995). MHC-dependent mate preferences in humans. *Proceedings of the Royal Society of London. Series B, Containing papers of a Biological character. Royal Society (Great Britain).* 260, 245–9.

85 More on **tickling oneself** in the article Weiskrantz, L., Elliott, J. & Darlington, C. (1971). Preliminary observations on tickling oneself. *Nature.* 230, 598–9. These observations have since been linked to consciousness in the article Cotterill, R. M. J. (1996). Prediction and internal feedback in conscious perception. *Journal of Consciousness Studies.* 3, 245–66. **Brain scanning of tickling** with and without a robotic arm: Blakemore, S.-J., Wolpert, D.-M. & Frith, C.-D. (1998). Central cancellation of self-produced tickle sensation. *Nature Neuroscience.* 1, 635–40.

86 Wilder Penfield's observations on **the homunculus** are described in Penfield, W. & Rasmussen, T. (1950). *The Cerebral Cortex of Man: A Clinical Study of Localization of Function.* New York, NY: Macmillan.

88 The **"what" and "where" visual pathways** were described in Goodale, M. A. & Milner, A. D. (1992). Separate visual pathways for perception and action. *Trends in neurosciences.* 15, 20–5.

89 The case of **local versus distributed object processing** in the visual cortices: Haxby, J. V., Gobbini, M. I., Furey, M. L., Ishai, A., Schouten, J. L. & Pietrini, P. (2001). Distributed and overlapping representations of faces and objects in ventral temporal cortex. *Science.* 293, 2425–30.

6 Memories

94 **Confabulation in normal life** is described in the elegant experiment Johansson, P., Hall, L., Sikstrom, S. & Olsson, A. (2005). Failure to detect mismatches between intention and outcome in a simple decision task. *Science.* 310, 116–9.

96 The case of **Shereshevsky** is described in the excellent monograph Luria, A. R. (1968). *The Mind of a Mnemonist.* Cambridge, Mass: Harvard University Press.

99 A good reference to the role of the **prefrontal cortex in memory**: Wagner, A. D., Bunge, S. A. & Badre, D. (2004). Cognitive control, semantic memory, and priming: Contributions from prefrontal cortex. In: *The Cognitive Neurosciences.* 3rd ed. Ed. M. S. Gazzaniga. Cambridge, MA: MIT Press.

99 More information about **synesthesia** can be found in Ramachandran, V. S. & Hubbard, E. M. (2003). Hearing colors, tasting shapes. *Scientific American,* April. **Brain imaging of color synesthesia** is described in Hubbard, E. M., Arman, A. C., Ramachandran, V. S. & Boynton, G. M. (2005). Individual differences among grapheme-color synesthetes: brain-behavior correlations. *Neuron.* 45, 975–85.

99 The first known **description of synesthesia**: "A studious blind man who had mightily beat his head about visible object, and made use of the explications of his books and friends, to understand those names of light and colors, which often came his way, betrayed one day that he now understood what scarlet signified. Upon which, his friend demanded what scarlet was? The blind man answered, it was like the sound of a trumpet." Locke, J. (1690). *An Essay Concerning Human Understanding [reprinted 1994] Book 3.* New York, NY: Prometheus Books.

100 The original paper on **synesthesia by Galton**: Galton, F. (1880). Visualised numerals. *Nature.* 21, 252–6.

101 Brain activity in a **blind synaesthete** is described in Hansen, P. C., Stevens, M., Kringelbach, M. L. & Blakemore, C. (2005). An MEG study of colored-hearing synaesthesia in a late-blind synaesthete. *Society for Neuroscience.* 640.21.

101 **Further information on synesthesia** can be found on the website, UK *Synesthesia Association*: [http://www.uksynaesthesia.com/].

103 The example with **remembering sweet words** is taken from the very readable book on memory Schacter, D. (1999). *Searching for Memory. The Brain, the Mind and the Past.* New York, NY: Basic Books.

103 **The limits of short-term memory** of between five and nine elements can be found in Miller, G. A. (1956). The magical number seven, plus or minus two: some limits on our capacity for processing information. *The Psychological Review.* 63, 81–97.

104 Brenda Milner has been instrumental in studying **the memory of HM**: Milner, B. (1966). Amnesia following operation on the temporal lobes. In: *Amnesia: Clinical, Psychological and Medicolegal Aspects.* Eds. C. W. M. Whitty & O. L. London: Zangwill. Butterworths.

105 **Morris' water maze** is described in Morris, R. (1984). Developments of a water-maze procedure for studying spatial learning in the rat. *Journal of Neuroscience Methods.* 11, 47–60.

107 **Consolidation of memory traces** is a very interesting research area and more information can be found in Nader, K., Schafe, G. E. & LeDoux, J. E. (2000). The labile nature of consolidation theory. *Nature Reviews Neuroscience.* 1, 216–9. The **link between consolidation and REM sleep** comes from the paper: Crick, F. H. C. & Mitchison, G. (1983). The function of dream sleep. *Nature.* 304, 111–4.

107 The role of the **medial orbitofrontal cortex in confabulation** is described in Schnider, A. (2003). Spontaneous confabulation and the adaptation of thought to ongoing reality. *Nature Reviews Neuroscience.* 4, 662–71.

7 Learning

113 The **story of Hardy and Ramanujan** is well told in the book Dehaene, S. (1997). *The Number Sense. How the Mind creates Mathematics.* Oxford: Oxford University Press.

114 For those **mathematically inclined:** $1729 = 1^3 + 12^3 = 10^3 + 9^3$

115 The book about all those **remarkable numbers** is Le Lionnais, F. (1983). *Nombres Remarquables.* Paris: Hermann.

115 The **functions of the parietal lobes** have been mapped in the article Simon, O., Mangin, J. F., Cohen, L., Le Bihan, D. & Dehaene, S. (2002). Topographical layout of hand, eye, calculation, and language-related areas in the human parietal lobe. *Neuron.* 33, 475–87.

117 **Shakespeare's counting monkeys** Rosenkrantz and MacDuff are described in the paper Brannon, E. M. & Terrace, H. S. (1998). Ordering of the numerosities 1 to 9 by monkeys. *Science.* 282, 746–9.

117 The **parietal cortex shows a topographical layout**: Simon, O., Mangin, J. F., Cohen, L., Le Bihan, D. & Dehaene, S. (2002). Topographical layout of hand, eye, calculation, and language-related areas in the human parietal lobe. *Neuron.* 33, 475–87.

119 For more **information on stuttering**, read the review Büchel, C. & Sommer, M. (2004). What causes stuttering? *PLoS Biology.* 2, E46. As well as the related paper: Sommer, M., Koch, M. A., Paulus, W., Weiller, C. & Büchel, C. (2002). Disconnection of speech-relevant brain areas in persistent developmental stuttering. *Lancet.* 360, 380–3.

120 **Stuttering across the whole life span** is described in Craig, A., Hancock, K., Tran, Y., Craig, M. & Peters, K. (2002). Epidemiology of stuttering in the community across the entire life span. *Journal of Speech, Language, and Hearing Research.* 45, 1097–105.

121 **The history of stuttering** has been described in the book Bobrick, B. (1995). *Knotted Tongues. Stuttering in History and the Quest for a Cure.* New York, NY: Simon & Schuster.

122 **Artificial stuttering** using sound delays can be found in a paper Lee, B. S. (1951). Artificial stutter. *The Journal of Speech and Hearing Disorders.* 16, 53–5.

123 An overview of the present **state-of-the-art of reading brain research** can be found in the book Cornelissen, P. L., Kringelbach, M. L., Pugh, K. & Hansen, P. C. (in press). *The Neural Basis of Reading.* New York, NY: Oxford University Press.

125 More information **on the visual word form area** can be found in Dehaene, S. (2003). Natural born readers. *New Scientist,* July 5, pp 30–3.

126 The classic **psychological paper on visual word forms**: Warrington, E. K. & Shallice, T. (1980). Word-form dyslexia. *Brain.* 103, 99–112. Since then the hunt is on for a **brain correlate of this psychological construct**: Cohen, L., Dehaene, S., Naccache, L., Lehericy, S., Dehaene-Lambertz, G., Henaff, M. A. & Michel, F. (2000). The visual word form area: spatial and temporal characterization of an initial stage of reading in normal subjects and posterior split-brain patients. *Brain.* 123, 291–307.

128 There is convergence of **Kanji and Kana in the brain**: Nakamura, K., Dehaene, S., Jobert, A., Le Bihan, D. & Kouider, S. (2005). Subliminal convergence of Kanji and Kana words: further evidence for functional parcellation of the posterior temporal cortex in visual word perception. *Journal of Cognitive Neuroscience.* 17, 954–68. However, some researchers are **not convinced by the data**: Price, C. J. & Devlin, J. T. (2003). The myth of the visual word form area. *Neuroimage.* 19, 473–81.

129 The idea of the **VWFA as a skill zone** is developed in Shaywitz, B. A., Shaywitz, S. E., Blachman, B. A., Pugh, K. R., Fulbright, R. K., Skudlarski, P., Mencl, W. E., Constable, R. T., Holahan, J. M., Marchione, K. E., Fletcher, J. M., Lyon, G. R. & Gore, J. C. (2004). Development of left occipitotemporal systems for skilled reading in children after a phonologically- based intervention. *Biological Psychiatry.* 55, 926–33.

129 The paper on the **dynamical development of reading using MEG**: Pammer, K., Hansen, P. C., Kringelbach, M. L., Holliday, I. E., Barnes, G. R., Hillebrand, A., Singh, K. D. & Cornelissen, P. L. (2004). Visual word recognition: The first half second. *Neuroimage.* 22, 1819–25.

131 **Localised representation of objects in the brain** has been described in the paper Hasson, U., Harel, M., Levy, I. & Malach, R. (2003). Large-scale mirror-symmetry organization of human occipito-temporal object areas. *Neuron.* 37, 1027–41.

134 **Fluid absorption** is akin the idea of "funktionslust" put forward in Bühler, K. (1927). *Die Krise der Psychologie.* Jena: Gustav Fischer.

135 The experiment using nursery **children and reward** was described in Lepper, M. R., Greene, D. & Nisbett, R. E. (1973). Undermining children's intrinsic interest with extrinsic reward: A test of the overjustification hypothesis. *Journal of Personality and Social Psychology.* 28, 129–37. More fundamental information on the **problems of oversimplified models of rewards and punishments**: McGraw, K. O. (1978). The detrimental effects of reward on performance: a literature review and a prediction model. In: *The Hidden Costs of Reward*, Eds. M. R. Lepper & D. Greene. Morristown, NJ: Lawrence Erlbaum.

8 Madness

140 Read more **on depression** in the excellent book Wolpert, L. (2000). *Malignant Sadness: The Anatomy of Depression.* London: Free Press.

142 The **meta-analysis of clinical studies of depression,** which has created much discussion: Kirsch, I. Deacon, B. J., Huedo-Medina, T. B., Scoboria, A., Moore, T. J., et al. (2008). Initial severity and antidepressant benefits: a meta-analysis of data submitted to the Food and Drug Administration. *PLoS Medicine.* 5(2), e45. doi:10.1371/journal.pmed.005004. Kirsch,

I. & Sapirstein, G. (1998). Listening to Prozac but hearing placebo: a meta-analysis of antidepressant medication. *Prevention and Treatment*. 1, 0002a. Since then Irving Kirsch has published other interesting papers: Kirsch, I. (2000). Are drug and placebo effects in depression additive? *Biological Psychiatry*. 47, 733–5. Kirsch, I. (2003). St John's wort, conventional medication, and placebo: An egregious double standard. *ComplementaryTtherapies in Medicine*. 11, 193–5. It is worth noticing that the pharmaceutical industry spends a lot of funds on research but that this also reaps enormous profit of which an ever larger percentage is used to market the drugs such antidepressants to the medical doctors who proscribe them. This leads to some **ethical considerations about depression and the pharmaceutical industry** as discussed on www.healthyskepticism.org.

142 Read more about the effectiveness of **antidepressants and placebo for children and adolescents** in the interesting articles Jureidini, J. N., Doecke, C. J., Mansfield, P. R., Haby, M. M., Menkes, D. B., & Tonkin, A. L. (2004). Efficacy and safety of antidepressants for children and adolescents. *BMJ*. 328, 879–83. Garland, E. J. (2004). Facing the evidence: Antidepressant treatment in children and adolescents. *CMAJ*. 170, 489–91.

143 The recent **recommendations regarding antidepressants** from the Food and Drugs Administration can be found on the website www.fda.gov/cder/drug/antidepressants/Antidepressanst-PHA.htm

144 Two studies are often cited concerning the role of the **subgenual cingulate cortex in depression**: Drevets, W. C., Price, J. L., Simpson, J. R., Jr., Todd, R. D., Reich, T., Vannier, M., & Raichle, M. E. (1997). Subgenual prefrontal cortex abnormalities in mood disorders. *Nature*. 386, 824–7. Mayberg, H. S., Brannan, S. K., & Mahurin (1997). Cingulate function in depression: A potential predictor of treatment response. *Neuroreport*. 8, 1057–61. The **resting network of the brain** has been described in two papers: Gusnard, D. A. & Raichle, M. E. (2001). Searching for a baseline: functional imaging and the resting human brain. *Nature Reviews Neuroscience*. 2, 685–94. Raichle, M. E., MacLeod, A. M., Snyder, A. Z., Powers, W. J., Gusnard, D. A., & Shulman, G. L. (2001). A default mode of brain function. *Proceedings of the National Academy of Sciences of the United States of America*. 98, 676–82. The activity in **neurons in the monkey brain** has been described in the article: Rolls, E. T., Inoue, K., & Browning, A. (2003). Activity of primate subgenual cingulate cortex neurons is related to sleep. *Journal of Neurophysiology*. 90, 134–42.

144 Mayberg has recently claimed remarkable results of **deep brain stimulation for depression**: Mayberg, H. S., Lozano, A. M., Voon, V., McNeely, H. E., Seminowicz, D., Hamani, C., Schwalb, J. M. & Kennedy, S. H. (2005). Deep brain stimulation for treatment-resistant depression. *Neuron*. 45, 651–60.

146 **Creativity, madness, and religion** are linked in the chapter Thornhill-Miller, B. (in press). Creativity, religion, and the extraordinary-ordinary theory of novelty and the numinous. In: *Handbook on the Psychology of Religion*, Ed. D. Wulff. Oxford: Oxford University Press.

146 Two very readable books exist on the **creation of the Oxford English Dictionary**: Winchester, S. (1999). *The Surgeon of Crowthorne: A Tale of Murder, Madness and the Oxford English Dictionary*. Oxford: Oxford University Press. Winchester, S. (2003). *The Meaning of Everything: The Story of the Oxford English Dictionary*. Oxford: Oxford University Press.

153 Tom Cullen's important findings of the number of **cells in the thalamus of schizophrenic brains** can be found in the paper Cullen, T. J., Walker, M. A., Parkinson, N., Craven, R., Crow, T. J., Esiri, M. M., & Harrison, P. J. (2003). A postmortem study of the mediodorsal nucleus of the thalamus in schizophrenia. *Schizophrenia Research*. 60, 157–66. Bente **Pakkenberg's original findings** are described in the article Pakkenberg, B. (1990). Pronounced reduction of total neuron number in mediodorsal thalamic nucleus and nucleus accumbens in schizophrenics. *Archives of General Psychiatry*. 47, 1023–8. Pakkenberg, B. (1992). The volume of the mediodorsal thalamic nucleus in treated and untreated schizophrenics. *Schizophrenia Research*. 7, 95–100.

154 Bentham outlined some of his **utilitarian ideas** in Bentham, J. (1789). *The Principles of Morals and Legislation*. London: T. Payne.

9 Stimulants

158 Two classical anthropological texts have, as mentioned earlier, described **food in cultural settings**: Douglas, M. (1966). *Purity and Danger : An Analysis of Concepts of Pollution and Taboo*. London: Routledge & Kegan Paul. Lévi-Strauss, C. (1964). *Le Cru et Le Cuit*. Paris: Librairie Plon.

159 Jared Diamond was awarded the Pulitzer Prize for his interesting book on **the history of the last 10,000 years of humanity**: Diamond, J. M. (1999). *Guns, Germs, and Steel: The Fates of Human Societies*. New York: Norton.

160 **The concept of qualia** is described in an interesting article by philosopher David Chalmers: Chalmers, D. (1995). Facing up to the problem of consciousness. *Journal of Consciousness Studies*. 2, 200–19.

160 Paul Rozin has written on **preferences for food intake** in the article Rozin, P. (2001). Food preference. In: *International Encyclopedia of the Social & Behavioral Sciences*. Eds. N. J. Smelser & P. B. Baltes. Amsterdam: Elsevier. pp. 5719–22. More information about **food intake and culture** can be found in the book: Kass, L. R. (1994). *The Hungry Soul: Eating and the Perfecting of Our Nature*. Chicago: University of Chicago Press.

166 I have written several reviews on what brain scanning experiments can tell us about **pleasure in general**: Kringelbach M. L. (2005). The human orbitofrontal cortex: linking reward to hedonic experience. *Nature Reviews Neuroscience*. 6, 691–702. Kringelbach, M. L. (2004). Food for thought: Hedonic experience beyond homeostasis in the human brain. *Neuroscience*. 126, 807–19. The details of our experiment on the **subjective experience of amphetamine** can be found in the following article: Völlm, B. A., de Araujo, I. E. T., Cowen, P. J., Rolls, E. T., Kringelbach, M. L., Smith, K. A., Jezzard, P., Heal, R. J. & Matthews, P. M. (2004). Methamphetamine activates reward circuitry in drug naïve human subjects. *Neuropsychopharmacology.* 29, 1715–22.

166 Good places to start reading about the **neuroimaging of pain** are the review articles Petrovic, P. & Ingvar, M. (2002). Imaging cognitive modulation of pain processing. *Pain.* 95, 1–5. Leknes, S. & Tracey, I. (2008). A common neurobiology for pain and pleasure. *Nature Reviews Neuroscience.* 9, 314–20.

167 **Michel de Montaigne's famous *Essays*** can be found in several volumes: Montaigne, M. (15801588). *Essais de Messire Michel Seigneur de Montaigne. 3 vols.* S. Millanges, Bourdeaux.

167 More details on the **placebo neuroimaging experiment** can be found in the article Petrovic, P., Kalso, E., Petersson, K. M. & Ingvar, M. (2002). Placebo and opioid analgesia—imaging a shared neuronal network. *Science.* 295, 1737–40.

168 A recent extensive **review on placebo** is the following: Colloca, L. & Benedetti, F. (2005). Placebos and painkillers: Is mind as real as matter? *Nature Reviews Neuroscience.* 6, 545–52.

173 The most **authoritative book on marijuana** is written by Leslie Iversen, who is professor of pharmacology in Oxford and Cambridge: Iversen, L. L. (2007). *The Science of Marijuana.* 2nd edition. Oxford: Oxford University Press. Another interesting **book on marijuana** is the following: Grinspoon, L. & Bakalar, J. B. (1997). *Marihuana, the Forbidden Medicine.* New Haven: Yale University Press.

174 **Marijuana as a cure for melancholia** was proposed by Robert Burton in his book Burton, R. (1621). *The Anatomy of Melancholy. [1989 version eds. T. C. Faulkner, N. K. Kiessling & R. L. Blair].* Oxford: Clarendon Press.

181 **The history of narcotic drugs** and the pursuit of oblivion are described in the book Davenport-Hines, R. (2002). *The Pursuit of Oblivion: A Global History of Narcotics.* London: W.W. Norton.

10 Sex

185 Read more about the fascinating behavior and **communication with infrasounds in elephants** in, Payne, K. (1998). *Silent Thunder. In the Presence of Elephants*. London: Allan Lane Press.

186 **Schwarz' original paper on the bonobo**: Schwarz, E. (1929). Das Vorkommen des Schimpansen auf den linken Kongo-Ufer. *Revue de zoologie et de botanique africaines* 16, 425–6.

186 The fascinating **life of bonobos** is entertainingly described in De Waal, F. B. M. & Lanting, F. (1997). *Bonobo: The Forgotten Ape*. Berkeley: University of California Press.

187 A very readable account of **Goodall's research** is described in her book Goodall, J. (1990). *Through a Window*. London: Weidenfeld & Nicholson.

188 The origin of the term **missionary position in the English language** comes from the book Malinowski, B. (1929) *The Sexual Life of Savages in North-Western Melanesia*. London: Routledge. The article on the use of **missionary position in bonobos**: Tratz, E. P. & Heck, H. (1954). Der afrikanische Anthropoide "Bonobo": Eine neue Menschenaffengattung. *Säugertierkundliche Mitteilungen* 2, 97–101.

188 The first reference to **orgasms in rhesus monkeys** can be found in Zumpe, D. & Michael, R. P. (1968). The clutching reaction and orgasm in the female rhesus monkey (*Macaca mulatta*). *The Journal of endocrinology*. 40, 117–23.

190 Jane **Goodall's research in chimpanzees** is deeply fascinating. A good source is Goodall, J. (1990). *Through a Window*. London: Weidenfeld & Nicholson.

190 **Kanzi's abilities** are described in Savage-Rumbaugh, S. & Lewin, R. (1994). *Kanzi: The ape at the Brink of the Human Mind*. New York: Wiley.

191 Gordon **Gallup's mirror test** was first described in Gallup, G. C. (1970). Chimpanzees: Self-recognition. *Science* 167, 86–7.

192 The **hominid fossil footprints** were found at Laetoli in Tanzania: Hay, R. L. & Leakey, M. D. (1982). Fossil footprints of Laetoli. *Scientific American* February, 50–7.

193 Alfred C. **Kinsey's original pioneering studies** can be found in two monumental volumes: Kinsey, A. C., Pomeroy, W. B., & Martin, C. E. (1948). *Sexual Behavior in the Human Male.* London, Philadelphia: W. Saunders. Kinsey, A. C. (1953). *Sexual Behavior in the Human Female.* London, Philadelphia: W. Saunders.

195 Two recently published **biographies on Kinsey** are the following, where the former is clearly the best: Gathorne-Hardy, J. (1998). *Alfred C. Kinsey: Sex the Measure of Things, a Biography.* London: Chatto & Windus. Jones, J. H. (1997). *Alfred C. Kinsey: A Public Private Life.* New York, NY; London: W.W. Norton.

197 More information on **phantom pain** can be found in the excellent article Melzack, R. (1992). Phantom limbs. *Scientific American.* 266, 120–6. **Other interesting information on phantom limbs** can be found in Ramachandran, V. S. & Rogers-Ramachandran, D. (2000). Phantom limbs and neural plasticity. *Archives of neurology.* 57, 317–20. Ramachandran, V. S. & Hirstein, W. (1998). The perception of phantom limbs. The D. O. Hebb lecture. *Brain.* 121, 1603–30.

200 The first report of combining **MEG and DBS for phantom limb pain** can be found in Kringelbach, M. L., Jenkinson, N., Green, A. L., Owen, S. L. F., Hansen, P. C., Cornelissen, P. L., Holliday, I. E., Stein, J. & Aziz, T. Z. (2007). Deep brain stimulation for chronic pain investigated with magnetoencephalography. *Neuroreport.* 8(3), 223–228.

201 Read more about the experiments on **curing phantom pain** in Ramachandran, V. S. & Rogers-Ramachandran, D. (1996). Synaesthesia in phantom limbs induced with mirrors. *Proceedings of the Royal Society of London. Series B, Biology. Royal Society (Great Britain).* 263, 377–86.

201 The **plasticity in musicians** is described in Munte, T. F., Altenmüller, E., & Jancke, L. (2002). The musician's brain as a model of neuroplasticity. *Nature Reviews Neuroscience.* 3, 473–8. **Plasticity in primary auditory cortex** is described in, Pantev, C., Ross, B., Fujioka, T., Trainor, L. J., Schulte, M., & Schulz, M. (2003). Music and learning-induced cortical plasticity. *Annals of the New York Academy of Sciences.* 999, 438–50.

201 **Neurogenesis later in life** is for example described in Gould, E., Reeves, A. J., Fallah, M., Tanapat, P., Gross, C. G. & Fuchs, E. (1999). Hippocampal neurogenesis in adult Old World primates. *Proceedings of the National Academy of Sciences of the United States of America.* 96, 5263–7.

202 The study of **humans having sex in a brain scanner** is described in Schultz, W. W., van Andel, P., Sabelis, I., & Mooyaart, E. (1999). Magnetic resonance imaging of male and female genitals during coitus and female sexual arousal. *BMJ.* 319, 1596–1600.

202 **Leonardo da Vinci's drawings of coitus** have probably belonged to Queen Victoria, as they belong to the drawings owned by the English monarchy: Clark, K. & Pedretti, C. (1968). *The drawings of Leonardo da Vinci in the Collection of Her Majesty the Queen at Windsor Castle.* London: Phaidon. It may not fit the official image of the queen and her times but we now know that she enjoyed marijuana. **Other anatomical drawings** of intercourse can be found in, Dickinson, R. (1949). *Human Sex Anatomy, a Topographical Hand Atlas.* 2nd edn. London: Baillière, Tindall & Cox. An important study of human sexuality is: Masters, W. & Johnson, V. (1966). *Human Sexual Response.* Boston, MA: Little & Brown.

204 There are only very few studies on sex in brain scanners. The most thorough **study on male orgasms** in brain scanners is Holstege, G., Georgiadis, J. R., Paans, A. M., Meiners, L. C., van der Graaf, F. H. & Reinders, A. A. (2003). Brain activation during human male ejaculation. *The Journal of neuroscience.* 23, 9185–93. And female orgasms: Two other studies exist but with **less convincing results**: Graber, B., Rohrbaugh, J. W., Newlin, D. B., Varner, J. L. & Ellingson, R. J. (1985). EEG during masturbation and ejaculation. *Archives of sexual behavior.* 14, 491–503. Tiihonen J., Kuikka J., Kupila J., Partanen K., Vainio P., Airaksinen J., Eronen M., Hallikainen T., Paanila J., Kinnunen I., & et al. (1994). Increase in cerebral blood flow of right prefrontal cortex in man during orgasm. *Neuroscience letters.* 170, 241–3.

204 The brain activity of **female orgasms** is described in Georgiadis, J. R., Kortekaas, R., Kuipers, R., Nieuwenburg, A., Pruim, J., Reinders, A. A. & Holstege, G. (2006). Regional cerebral blood flow changes associated with clitorally induced orgasm in healthy women. *The European journal of neuroscience.* 24, 3305–16.

205 Two experiments investigated the **neural correlates of erotic photos**: Redouté J., Stoléru S., Grégoire M. C., Costes N., Cinotti L., Lavenne F., Le Bars D., Forest M. G., & Pujol J. F. (2000). Brain processing of visual sexual stimuli in human males. *Human Brain Mapping.* 11, 162–177. Hamann S., Herman R. A., Nolan C. L., & Wallen K. (2004). Men and women differ in amygdala response to visual sexual stimuli. *Nature neuroscience.* 7, 411–6.

205 Monkeys will **pay to view** red perineums and higher ranking monkeys: Deaner, R. O., Khera, A. V. & Platt, M. L. (2005). Monkeys pay per view: Adaptive valuation of social images by rhesus macaques. *Current biology.* 15, 543–8.

208 Some have argued for fundamental **differences between the male and female brain**: Cahill, L. (2006). Why sex matters for neuroscience. *Nature Reviews Neuroscience.* 7, 477–84.

209 Some claim to have found **romantic love in the brain**: Bartels, A. & Zeki, S. (2000). The neural basis of romantic love. *Neuroreport.* 11, 3829–34.

11 Future Considerations

212 Daniel Kahneman described his **happiness findings** in two papers: Kahneman, D., Krueger, A. B., Schkade, D. A., Schwarz, N. & Stone, A. A. (2004). A survey method for characterizing daily life experience: The day reconstruction method. *Science.* 306, 1776–80. Kahneman, D., Krueger, A. B., Schkade, D., Schwarz, N. & Stone, A. A. (2006). Would you be happier if you were richer? A focusing illusion. *Science.* 312, 1908–10.

219 Bentham outlined some of his **utilitarian ideas** in Bentham, J. (1789). *The Principles of Morals and Legislation.* London: T. Payne.

224 One of the most autoritative sources on **population growth** is the book Cohen, J. E. (1995). *How Many People Can the Earth Support?* New York, NY: W.W. Norton. The estimate of the upper limit is taken from the article: Gowdy, J. M. & McDaniel, C. N. (1995). One world, one experiment: Addressing the biodiversity-economics conflict. *Ecological Economics.* 15, 181–92.

225 **Affective forecasting** is entertainingly described in Gilbert, D. (2006). *Stumbling on Happiness.* New York, NY: Random House.

226 Dyson's idea on **different time scales** is described in the book Dyson, F. (1989). *Infinite In All Directions.* New York, NY: Harper.

BIBLIOGRAPHY

Akelaitis, A. J. (1944). A study of gnosis, praxis, and language following section of the corpus callosum. *Journal of Neurosurgery*, 1, 94–102.

Aserinsky, E. & Kleitman, N. (1953). Regularly occurring periods of eye motility and concomitant phenomena during sleep. *Science*, 118, 273–274.

Balick, M. J. & Cox, P. A. (1996). *Plants, People, and Culture. The Science of Etnobotany.* New York, NY: W H Freeman.

Bartels, A. & Zeki, S. (2000). The neural basis of romantic love. *Neuroreport*, 11, 3829–3834.

Bear, M. F., Connors, B. W. & Paradiso, M. A. (2006). *Neuroscience. Exploring the Brain. 3rd ed.* New York, NY: Lippincott, Williams & Wilkins.

Bechara, A., Damasio, A. R., Damasio, H. & Anderson, S. W. (1994). Insensitivity to future consequences following damage to human prefrontal cortex. *Cognition*, 50, 7–15.

Bentham, J. (1789). *The Principles of Morals and Legislation.* London: T. Payne.

Berger, H. (1929). Über das Elektroenkephalogramm des Menschen. *Archiv für Psychiatrie und Nervenkrankeiten*, 87, 527–570.

Berkeley, G. (1709). *An Essay Towards a New Theory of Vision*: Dublin: Pepyat.

Berridge, K. C. (1996). Food reward: Brain substrates of wanting and liking. *Neuroscience and Biobehavioral Reviews*, 20, 1–25.

Berridge K. C. & Kringelbach M. L. (2008). Affective neuroscience of pleasure: Reward in humans and animals. *Psychopharmacology,* 199, 457–480.

Bigelow, H. J. (1850). Dr. Harlow's case of recovery from the passage of an iron bar through the head. *The American Journal of the Medical Sciences,* 20, 13–22.

Bindra, D. (1978). How adaptive behavior is produced: A perceptual-motivational alternative to response-reinforcement. *Behavioral and Brain Sciences,* 1, 41–91.

Blakemore, S.-J., Wolpert, D.-M. & Frith, C.-D. (1998). Central cancellation of self-produced tickle sensation. *Nature Neuroscience,* 1, 635–640.

Blum, D. (2002). *Love at Goon Park: Harry Harlow and the Science of Affection.* New York, NY: Perseus Publishing.

Bobrick, B. (1995). *Knotted Tongues. Stuttering in History and the Quest for a Cure.* New York, NY: Simon & Schuster.

Boole, G. (1854). *An Investigation of the Laws of Thought on Which Are Founded the Mathematical Theories of Logic and Probabilities.* Cambridge: Macmillan and Co.

Borges, J. L. (1944). *Ficciones.* New York, NY: Weidenfeld.

Brand, S. (1999). *The Clock of the Long Now: Time and Responsibility.* New York, NY: Basic Books.

Brannon, E. M. & Terrace, H. S. (1998). Ordering of the numerosities 1 to 9 by monkeys. *Science,* 282, 746–749.

Broca, M. P. (1861). Remarques sur le siége de la faculté du langage articulé, suivies d'une observation d'aphémie (perte de la parole). *Bulletin de la Société Anatomique,* 6, 330–357.

Broca, P. (1878). Anatomie comparée des circonvolutions cérébrales: Le grand lobe limbique et le scissure limbique dans la série des mammifères. *Rev d'Anthrop Par,* 3.s, 385–498.

Brodmann, K. (1909). *Vergleichende Lokalisationslehre der Grosshirnrinde in ihren Prinzipien dargestellt auf Grund des Zellenbaues.* Leipzig: Barth.

Brown, D. E. (1991). *Human Universals.* New York, NY: McGraw-Hill.

Bruce, V. & Young, A. (1986). Understanding face recognition. *British Journal of Psychology (London, England),* 77, 305–327.

Buchel, C. & Sommer, M. (2004). What causes stuttering? *PLoS Biology,* 2, E46.

Bühler, K. (1927). *Die Krise der Psychologie.* Jena: Gustav Fischer.

Burkert, W. (1996). *Creation of the Sacred. Tracks of Biology in Early Religions.* Cambridge, MA: Harvard University Press.

Burton, R. (1621). *The Anatomy of Melancholy. [1989 version eds. T. C. Faulkner, N. K. Kiessling & R. L. Blair].* Oxford: Clarendon Press.

Cabanac, M. (1971). Physiological role of pleasure. *Science,* 173, 1103–1107.

Cahill, L. (2006). Why sex matters for neuroscience. *Nature Reviews Neuroscience,* 7, 477–484.

Cannon, W. B. (1927). The James–Lange theory of Emotion. *American Journal of Psychology,* 39, 106–124.

Caton, R. (1875). The electrical currents of the brain. *British Medical Journal,* 1, 278.

Chalmers, D. (1995). Facing up to the problem of consciousness. *Journal of Consciousness Studies,* 2, 200–219.

Clark, K. & Pedretti, C. (1968). *The Drawings of Leonardo da Vinci In the Collection of Her Majesty the Queen at Windsor Castle.* London: Phaidon.

Cohen, D. (1968). Magnetoencephalography: Evidence of magnetic fields produced by alpha-rhythm currents. *Science,* 161, 784–786.

Cohen, D. (1970). Detection of magnetic fields outside the human head produced by alpha rhythm currents. *Electroencephalography and Clinical Neurophysiology,* 28, 102.

Cohen, J. E. (1995). *How Many People Can the Earth Support?* New York, NY: W. W. Norton.

Cohen, L., Dehaene, S., Naccache, L., Lehericy, S., Dehaene-Lambertz, G., Henaff, M. A., et al. (2000). The visual word form area: Spatial and temporal characterization of an initial stage of reading in normal subjects and posterior split-brain patients. *Brain,* 123, 291–307.

Colloca, L. & Benedetti, F. (2005). Placebos and painkillers: Is mind as real as matter? *Nature Reviews Neuroscience,* 6, 545–552.

Cornelissen, P. L., Kringelbach, M. L., Pugh, K. & Hansen, P. C. (in press). *The Neural Basis of Reading.* New York, NY: Oxford University Press.

Cotterill, R. M. J. (1996). Prediction and internal feedback in conscious perception. *Journal of Consciousness Studies,* 3, 245–266.

Cotterill, R. M. J. (1998). *Enchanted Looms. Conscious Networks in Brains and Computers.* Cambridge: Cambridge University Press.

Craig, A. D. (2002). Opinion: How do you feel? Interoception: The sense of the physiological condition of the body. *Nature Reviews Neuroscience,* 3, 655–666.

Craig, A., Hancock, K., Tran, Y., Craig, M. & Peters, K. (2002). Epidemiology of stuttering in the community across the entire life span. *Journal of Speech, Language, and Hearing Research,* 45, 1097–1105.

Crick, F. & Mitchison, G. (1983). The function of dream sleep. *Nature,* 304, 111–114.

Cullen, T. J., Walker, M. A., Parkinson, N., Craven, R., Crow, T. J., Esiri, M. M., et al. (2003). A postmortem study of the mediodorsal nucleus of the thalamus in schizophrenia. *Schizophrenia Research,* 60, 157–166.

Damasio, A. R. (1994). *Descartes' Error.* New York: Putnam.

Darwin, C. (1859). *The Origin of Species by Means of Natural Selection, or, the Preservation of Favoured Races in the Struggle for Life.* London: John Murray.

Darwin, C. (1872). *The Expression of the Emotions in Man and Animals.* Chicago, IL: University of Chicago Press.

Darwin, C. & Wallace, A. (1858). On the tendency of species to form varieties; and on the perpetuation of varieties and species by natural means of selection. *Journal of the Proceedings of the Linnean Society, Zoology,* 3, 45–62.

Davenport-Hines, R. (2002). *The Pursuit of Oblivion: A Global History of Narcotics.* London: W.W. Norton.

Davis, W. (1996). *One River. Explorations and Discoveries in the Amazon Rain Forest.* New York, NY: Simon & Schuster.

Dawkins, R. (1976). *The Selfish Gene.* Oxford University Press: Oxford.

Dawkins, R. (2006). *The God Delusion*. London: Bantam Books.

De Araujo, I. E. T., Kringelbach, M. L., Rolls, E. T. & Hobden, P. (2003). The representation of umami taste in the human brain. *Journal of Neurophysiology*, 90, 313–319.

de Waal, F. B. M. (1997). *Good Natured. The Origins of Right and Wrong in Humans and Oher Animals*. Cambridge, Mass: Harvard University Press.

de Waal, F. B. M. & Lanting, F. (1997). *Bonobo: The Forgotten Ape*. University of Berkeley: California Press.

Deaner, R. O., Khera, A. V. & Platt, M. L. (2005). Monkeys pay per view: Adaptive valuation of social images by rhesus macaques. *Current Biology*, 15, 543–548.

Dehaene, S. (1997). *The Number Sense. How the Mind creates Mathematics*. Oxford University Press: Oxford.

Dehaene, S. (2003). Natural born readers. *NewScientist*, pp 30–33.

Descartes, R. (1649). *Les Passions de l'âme*. Paris: Henry LeGras.

Diamond, J. M. (1999). *Guns, Germs, and Steel: The Fates of Human Societies*. New York, NY: Norton.

Dickinson, R. (1949). *Human Sex Anatomy, a Topographical Hand Atlas. 2nd ed*. London: Baillière, Tindall & Cox.

Dolan, R. J., Fink, G. R., Rolls, E., Booth, M., Holmes, A., Frackowiak, R. S., et al. (1997). How the brain learns to see objects and faces in an impoverished context. *Nature*, 389, 596–599.

Douglas, M. (1966). *Purity and Danger: An Analysis of Concepts of Pollution and Taboo*. London: Routledge & Kegan Paul.

Drevets, W. C., Price, J. L., Simpson, J. R., Jr., Todd, R. D., Reich, T., Vannier, M., et al. (1997). Subgenual prefrontal cortex abnormalities in mood disorders. *Nature*, 386, 824–827.

Dutton, D. G. & Aron, A. P. (1974). Some evidence for heightened sexual attraction under conditions of high anxiety. *Journal of Personality and Social Psychology*, 30, 510–517.

Duvernoy, M. (1999). *Human Brain Atlas. 2nd ed*. New York, NY: Springer-Verlag.

Duyme, M., Dumaret, A. C. & Tomkiewicz, S. (1999). How can we boost IQs of "dull children"?: A late adoption study. *Proceedings of the National Academy of Sciences of the United States of America*, 96, 8790–8794.

Dyson, F. (1989). *Infinite In All Directions*. New York, NY: Harper.

Eccles, J. C. & Gibson, W. C. (1979). *Sherrington. His Life and Thought*. New York, NY: Springer.

Ekman, P. (1982). *Emotion in the Human Face*. Cambridge: Cambridge University Press.

Ekman, P. & Davidson, R. J. (1994). *The Nature of Emotion: Fundamental Questions*. New York, NY: Oxford University Press.

Ekman, P. & Friesen, W.-V. (1971). Constants across cultures in the face and emotion. *Journal of Personality and Social Psychology*, 17(2), 124–129.

Flynn, J. R. (1984). The mean IQ of Americans: Massive gains 1932 to 1978. *Psychological Bulletin*, 95, 29–51.

Frijda, N. E. (2006). *The Laws of Emotion*. New York: Lawrence Erlbaum Associates.

Gallup, G. G. (1970). Chimpanzees: Self-recognition. *Science*, 167, 86–87.

Galton, F. (1880). Visualised numerals. *Nature*, 21, 252–256.

Garland, E. J. (2004). Facing the evidence: Antidepressant treatment in children and adolescents. *CMAJ*, 170, 489–491.

Gathorne-Hardy, J. (1998). *Alfred C. Kinsey: Sex the Measure of Things, a Biography*. London: Chatto & Windus.

Gazzaniga, M. (2004). *The New Cognitive Neurosciences. 3rd ed.* Cambridge, MA: MIT Press.

Gazzaniga, M. S. (1970). *The Bisected Brain*. New York, NY: Appleton-Century-Crofts.

Gazzaniga, M. S. (2005). Forty-five years of split-brain research and still going strong. *Nature Reviews Neuroscience*, 6, 653–659.

Gazzaniga, M. S. & LeDoux, J. E. (1978). *The Integrated Mind*. New York, NY: Plenum Press.

Gazzaniga, M. S. & Sperry, R. W. (1967). Language after section of the cerebral commissures. *Brain*, 90, 131–148.

Geake, J. G. & Hansen, P. C. (2005). Neural correlates of intelligence as revealed by fMRI of fluid analogies. *Neuroimage*, 26, 555–564.

Georgiadis, J. R., Kortekaas, R., Kuipers, R., Nieuwenburg, A., Pruim, J., Reinders, A. A., et al. (2006). Regional cerebral blood flow changes associated with clitorally induced orgasm in healthy women. *The European Journal of Neuroscience, 24*, 3305–3316.

Gilbert, D. (2006). *Stumbling on Happiness*. New York, NY: Random House.

Goodale, M. A. & Milner, A. D. (1992). Separate visual pathways for perception and action. *Trends in Neurosciences*, 15, 20–25.

Goodall, J. (1990). *Through A Window*. London: Weidenfeld & Nicholson.

Gould, E., Reeves, A. J., Fallah, M., Tanapat, P., Gross, C. G. & Fuchs, E. (1999). Hippocampal neurogenesis in adult Old World primates. *Proceedings of the National Academy of Sciences of the United States of America*, 96, 5263–5267.

Gowdy, J. M. & McDaniel, C. N. (1995). One world, one experiment: Addressing the biodiversity-economics conflict. *Ecological Economics*, 15, 181–192.

Graber, B., Rohrbaugh, J. W., Newlin, D. B., Varner, J. L. & Ellingson, R. J. (1985). EEG during masturbation and ejaculation. *Archives of Sexual Behavior*, 14, 491–503.

Gray, J. A. (1979). *Ivan Pavlov*. New York, NY: Viking Press.

Gray, J. R. & Thompson, P. M. (2004). Neurobiology of intelligence: Science and ethics. *Nature Reviews Neuroscience*, 5, 471–482.

Gregory, R. L. (1997). *Mirrors In Mind*. New York, NY: W. H. Freeman.

Gregory, R. L. (2004). *The Oxford Companion to the Mind. 2nd ed.* Oxford: Oxford University Press.

Grinspoon, L. & Bakalar, J. B. (1997). *Marihuana, the Forbidden Medicine*. New Haven, CT: Yale University Press.

Gusnard, D. A. & Raichle, M. E. (2001). Searching for a baseline: Functional imaging and the resting human brain. *Nature Reviews Neuroscience*, 2, 685–694.

Hamann, S., Herman, R. A., Nolan, C. L. & Wallen, K. (2004). Men and women differ in amygdala response to visual sexual stimuli. *Nature Neuroscience*, 7, 411–416.

Hansen, P. C., Stevens, M., Kringelbach, M. L. & Blakemore, C. (2005). An MEG study of colored-hearing synaesthesia in a late-blind synaesthete (Abstract). *Society for Neuroscience*, 640.21.

Harlow, H. F. (1958). The nature of love. *The American Psychologist,* 13, 673–685.

Harlow, J. (1868). Recovery after severe injury to the head. *Massachusetts Medical Society Publications,* 2, 327–347.

Harlow, J. M. (1848). Passage of an iron rod through the head. *Boston Medical and Surgical Journal,* 39, 389–393.

Hassin, R., Uleman, J. & Bargh, J. (2005). *The New Unconscious.* New York, NY: Oxford University Press.

Hasson, U., Harel, M., Levy, I. & Malach, R. (2003). Large-scale mirror-symmetry organization of human occipito-temporal object areas. *Neuron,* 37, 1027–1041.

Hauser, M. D. (1996). *The Evolution of Communication.* Cambridge, MA: MIT Press.

Haxby, J. V., Gobbini, M. I., Furey, M. L., Ishai, A., Schouten, J. L. & Pietrini, P. (2001). Distributed and overlapping representations of faces and objects in ventral temporal cortex. *Science,* 293, 2425–2430.

Hay, R. L. & Leakey, M. D. (1982). Fossil footprints of Laetoli. *Scientific American,* 246, 50–57.

Heath, R. G. (1963). Electrical Self-Stimulation of the Brain in Man. *The American Journal of Psychiatry,* 120, 571–577.

Hebb, D. O. (1949). *Organization of Behaviour: A Neuropsychological Theory. Stimulus and Response—and What Occurs in the Brain in the Interval between Them.* New York: Wiley.

Helenius, P., Tarkiainen, A., Cornelissen, P., Hansen, P. C. & Salmelin, R. (1999). Dissociation of normal feature analysis and deficient processing of letter-strings in dyslexic adults. *Cerebral Cortex (New York, N.Y.),* 9, 476–483.

Herrnstein, R. J. & Murray, C. (1994). *Bell Curve: Intelligence and Class Structure in American Life.* New York, NY: Free Press.

Hodgkin, A. L. & Huxley, A. F. (1952). A quantitative description of membrane current and its application to conduction and excitation in nerve. *The Journal of Physiology (London),* 117, 500–544.

Hölldobler, B. & Wilson, E. O. (1990). *The Ants.* Cambridge, MA: Belknap Press.

Holstege, G., Georgiadis, J. R., Paans, A. M., Meiners, L. C., van der Graaf, F. H. & Reinders, A. A. (2003). Brain activation during human male ejaculation. *The Journal of Neuroscience, 23*, 9185–9193.

Hopfield, J. (1982). Neural networks and physical systems with emergent collective computational abilities. *Proceedings of the National Academy of Sciences of the United States of America, 79*, 2254–2258.

Hubbard, E. M., Arman, A. C., Ramachandran, V. S. & Boynton, G. M. (2005). Individual differences among grapheme-color synesthetes: Brain-behavior correlations. *Neuron, 45*, 975–985.

Huettel, S. A., Song, A. W. & McCarthy, G. (2004). *Functional Magnetic Resonance Imaging*. Sunderland, MA: Sinauer.

Hull, C. L. (1951). *Essentials of Behavior*. New Haven, CT: Yale University Press.

Ingvar, D. H. & Risberg, J. (1965). Influence of mental activity upon regional cerebral blood flow in man. A preliminary study. *Acta neurologica Scandinavica. Supplementum, 14*, 183–186.

Iversen, L. L. (2000). *The Science of Marijuana*. Oxford: Oxford University Press.

Iversen, S. D. & Mishkin, M. (1970). Perseverative interference in monkeys following selective lesions of the inferior prefrontal convexity. *Experimental Brain Research, 11*, 376–386.

James, W. (1890). *The Principles of Psychology*. New York, NY: Henry Holt.

Jamison, K. R. (1995). *An Unquiet Mind. A Memoir of Moods and Madness*. New York, NY: Alfred A. Knopf.

Jezzard, P., Matthews, P. M. & Smith, S. M. (2001). *Functional MRI: An introduction to methods*. Oxford: Oxford University Press.

Johansson, P., Hall, L., Sikstrom, S. & Olsson, A. (2005). Failure to detect mismatches between intention and outcome in a simple decision task. *Science, 310*, 116–119.

Jones, J. H. (1997). *Alfred C. Kinsey: A Public Private Life*. New York; London: W. W. Norton.

Jureidini, J. N., Doecke, C. J., Mansfield, P. R., Haby, M. M., Menkes, D. B. & Tonkin, A. L. (2004). Efficacy and safety of antidepressants for children and adolescents. *BMJ*, 328, 879–883.

Kahneman, D., Diener, E. & Schwarz, M. (2003). *Well-Being: The Foundations of Hedonic Psychology*. New York, NY: Russell Sage Foundation.

Kahneman, D. & Tversky, A. (1979). Prospect Theory: An analysis of decision under risk. *Econometrica*, XLVII, 263–291.

Kahneman, D., Krueger, A. B., Schkade, D. A., Schwarz, N. & Stone, A. A. (2004). A survey method for characterizing daily life experience: The day reconstruction method. *Science*, 306, 1776–1780.

Kahneman, D., Krueger, A. B., Schkade, D., Schwarz, N. & Stone, A. A. (2006). Would you be happier if you were richer? A focusing illusion. *Science*, 312, 1908–1910.

Kandel, E. R., Schwartz, J. H. & Jessell, T. M. (2000). *Principles of Neural Science 4th ed*. New York, NY: McGraw-Hill.

Kanwisher, N., McDermott, J. & Chun, M. M. (1997). The fusiform face area: A module in human extrastriate cortex specialized for face perception. *The Journal of Neuroscience*, 17, 4302–4311.

Kass, L. R. (1994). *The Hungry Soul: Eating and the Perfecting of Our Nature*. Chicago: University of Chicago Press.

Kinsey, A. C. (1953). *Sexual Behavior in the Human Female*. Philadelphia; London: Saunders.

Kinsey, A. C., Pomeroy, W. B. & Martin, C. E. (1948). *Sexual Behavior in the Human Male*. W. Philadelphia; London: Saunders.

Kirsch, I. (2000). Are drug and placebo effects in depression additive? *Biological Psychiatry*, 47, 733–735.

Kirsch, I. (2003). St John's wort, conventional medication, and placebo: An egregious double standard. *Complementary Therapies in Medicine*, 11, 193–195.

Kirsch, I. & Sapirstein, G. (1998). Listening to Prozac but hearing Placebo: A meta-analysis of antidepressant medication. *Prevention and Treatment*, 1, 0002a.

Kirsch, I., Deacon, B. J., Huedo-Medina, T. B., Scoboria, A., Moore, T. J. & Johnson, B. T. (2008). Initial severity and antidepressant benefits: A metaanalysis of data submitted to the Food and Drug Administration. *PLoS Medicine*, 5, e45.

Konner, M. (2002). *The Tangled Wing: Biological Constraints on the Human Spirit. 2nd. ed.* New York, NY: Henry Holt.

Kornhuber, H. H. & Deecke, L. (1965). Hirnpotentialänderungen bei Willkürbewegungen und passiven Bewegungen des Menschen: Bereitschaftspotential und reafferente Potentiale. *Pflûgers Arch,* 284, 1–17.

Kringelbach, M. L. (2004a). Emotion. In R. L. Gregory (Ed.), *The Oxford Companion to the Mind 2nd ed* (pp. 287–290). Oxford: Oxford University Press.

Kringelbach, M. L. (2004b). Food for thought: Hedonic experience beyond homeostasis in the human brain. *Neuroscience,* 126, 807–819.

Kringelbach, M. L. (2004c). *Hjernerum. Den følelsesfulde hjerne.* København: People'sPress (med støtte fra Learning Lab Denmark).

Kringelbach, M. L. (2005). The orbitofrontal cortex: Linking reward to hedonic experience. *Nature Reviews Neuroscience,* 6, 691–702.

Kringelbach, M. L. & Berridge, K. C. (2008). *Pleasures of the Brain.* New York, NY: Oxford University Press.

Kringelbach, M. L., de Araujo, I. E. T. & Rolls, E. T. (2004). Taste-related activity in the human dorsolateral prefrontal cortex. *Neuroimage,* 21, 781–788.

Kringelbach, M. L. & Engell, A. (1997). Early development and plasticity in the brain. *Psyke & Logos,* 18, 266–286.

Kringelbach, M. L., Jenkinson, N., Green, A. L., Owen, S. L. F., Hansen, P. C., Cornelissen, P. L., et al. (2007). Deep brain stimulation for chronic pain investigated with magnetoencephalography. *Neuroreport,* 8(3), 223–228.

Kringelbach, M. L., Jenkinson, N., Owen, S. L. F. & Aziz, T. Z. (2007). Translational principles of deep brain stimulation. *Nature Reviews Neuroscience,* 8, 623–635.

Kringelbach, M. L., Lehtonen, A., Squire, S., Harvey, A., Craske, M. G., Holliday, I. E., et al. (2008). A specific and rapid neural signature for parental instinct. *PLoS ONE,* 3(2), e1664.

Kringelbach, M. L., O'Doherty, J., Rolls, E. T. & Andrews, C. (2003). Activation of the human orbitofrontal cortex to a liquid food stimulus is correlated with its subjective pleasantness. *Cerebral Cortex,* 13, 1064–1071.

Kringelbach, M. L. & Rolls, E. T. (2003). Neural correlates of rapid context-dependent reversal learning in a simple model of human social interaction. *Neuroimage,* 20, 1371–1383.

Kringelbach, M. L. & Rolls, E. T. (2004). The functional neuroanatomy of the human orbitofrontal cortex: Evidence from neuroimaging and neuropsychology. *Progress in Neurobiology,* 72, 341–372.

Krynauw, R. (1950). Infantile hemiplegia treated by removing one cerebral hemisphere. *Developmental Medicine and Child Neurology,* 28, 251–258.

Kwong, K. K., Belliveau, J. W., Chesler, D. A., Goldberg, I. E., Weisskoff, R. M., Poncelet, B. P., et al. (1992). Dynamic magnetic resonance imaging of human brain activity during primary sensory stimulation. *Proceedings of the National Academy of Sciences of the United States of America,* 89, 5675–5679.

Laland, K. N. & Brown, G. (2002). *Sense and Nonsense: Evolutionary Perspectives on Human Behaviour.* New York, NY: Oxford University Press.

Lange, C. G. (1887). Leipzig: *Über Gemüstbewegungen (Org. Om Sindsbevægelser).*

Lavie, P. (1996). *The Enchanted World of Sleep.* New Haven, CT: Yale University Press.

Le Lionnais, F. (1983). *Nombres remarquables.* Hermann: Paris.

LeDoux, J. E. (1996). *The Emotional Brain.* New York, NY: Simon and Schuster.

Lee, B. S. (1951). Artificial stutter. *The Journal of Speech and Hearing Disorders,* 16, 53–55.

Leknes, S. & Tracey, I. (2008). A common neurobiology for pain and pleasure. *Nature Reviews Neuroscience,* 9, 314–320.

Lepper, M. R. & Greene, D. (1978). *The Hidden Costs of Reward.* Morristown, NJ: Lawrence Erlbaum.

Lepper, M. R., Greene, D. & Nisbett, R. E. (1973). Undermining children's intrinsic interest with extrinsic reward: A test of the overjustification hypothesis. *Journal of Personality and Social Psychology,* 28, 129–137.

Lévi-Strauss, C. (1964). *Le Cru et Le Cuit. [1969] [The Raw and the Cooked: Introduction to a Science of Mythology. Jonathan Cape, London]*. Paris: Librairie Plon.

Lewin, R. (1998). *The Origin of Modern Humans*. New York, NY: W H Freeman & Co.

Lewis-Williams, D. (2002). *The Mind in the Cave: Consciousness and the Origins of Art*. London: Thames & Hudson.

Libet, B., Gleason, C. A., Wright, E. W. & Pearl, D. K. (1983). Time of conscious intention to act in relation to onset of cerebral activity (readiness-potential). The unconscious initiation of a freely voluntary act. *Brain*, 106, 623–642.

Locke, J. (1690). *An Essay Concerning Human Understanding [genoptrykt 1994]*. New York, NY: Prometheus Books.

Logothetis, N. K., Pauls, J., Augath, M., Trinath, T. & Oeltermann, A. (2001). Neurophysiological investigation of the basis of the fMRI signal. *Nature*, 412, 150–157.

Luria, A. R. (1968). *The Mind of a Mnemonist: A Little Book about a Vast Memory*. Cambridge, MA: Harvard University Press.

Machiavelli, N. (1513/1532 [1998]). *Il principe [The Prince]*. London: Penguin.

Mackintosh, A. R. (1988). Dr. Atanasoff's Computer. *Scientific American*, 259, 90–96.

MacLean, P. (1949). Psychosomatic disease and the "visceral brain": Recent developments bearing on the Papez theory of emotion. *Psychosomatic Medicine*, 11, 338–353.

MacLean, P. (1990). *The Triune Brain in Evolution*. New York, NY: Plenum Press.

Macmillan, M. (2000). *An Odd Kind of Fame: Stories of Phineas Gage*. Cambridge, MA: MIT Press.

Malinowski, B. (1929). *The Sexual Life of Savages in North-Western Melanesia*. London: Routledge.

Mansfield, P. (1977). Multi-planar image formation using NMR spin echoes. *Journal of Physical Chemistry*, 10, L55–58.

Martin, J. H. (1996). *Neuroanatomy. Text and Atlas*. New York: McGraw-Hill.

Masters, W. & Johnson, V. (1966). *Human sexual response*. Boston, MA: Little & Brown.

Mayberg, H. S., Brannan, S. K. & Mahurin (1997). Cingulate function in depression: A potential predictor of treatment response. *Neuroreport,* 8, 1057–1061.

Mayberg, H. S., Lozano, A. M., Voon, V., McNeely, H. E., Seminowicz, D., Hamani, C., et al. (2005). Deep brain stimulation for treatment-resistant depression. *Neuron,* 45, 651–660.

McCulloch, W. S. & Pitts, W. H. (1943). A logical calculus of the ideas immanent in nervous activity. *Bulletin of Mathematical Biology,* 5, 115–133.

McGraw, K. O. (1978). The detrimental effects of reward on performance: A literature review and a prediction model. In M. R. Lepper & D. Greene (Eds.), *The Hidden Costs of Reward.* Morristown, NJ: Lawrence Erlbaum.

McLeod, P., Heywood, C., Driver, J. & Zihl, J. (1989). Selective deficit of visual search in moving displays after extrastriate damage. *Nature,* 339, 466–467.

Melzack, R. (1992). Phantom limbs. *Scientific American,* 266, 120–126.

Miller, G. A. (1956). The magical number seven, plus or minus two: Some limits on our capacity for processing information. *The Psychological Review,* 63, 81–97.

Miller, J. (1998). *On Reflection.* London: National Gallery Publications.

Milner, B. (1966). Amnesia following operation on the temporal lobes. In C. W. M. Whitty & O. L. Zangwill (Eds.), *Amnesia: Clinical, Psychological and Medicolegal Aspects.* London: Butterworths.

Mithen, S. (1996). *The Prehistory of the Mind. A Search for the Origins of Art, Religion and Science.* London: Thames & Hudson.

Montaigne, M. D. (1580–1588). *Essais de Messire Michel Seigneur de Montaigne. 3 vols.* Bourdeaux: S. Millanges.

Monti-Bloch, L., Jennings-White, C. & Berliner, D. L. (1998). The human vomeronasal system. A review. *Annals of the New York Academy of Sciences,* 855, 373–389.

Morris, R. (1984). Developments of a water-maze procedure for studying spatial learning in the rat. *Journal of Neuroscience Methods,* 11, 47–60.

Munte, T. F., Altenmuller, E.& Jancke, L. (2002). The musician's brain as a model of neuroplasticity. *Nature Reviews Neuroscience,* 3, 473–478.

Nader, K., Schafe, G. E. & LeDoux, J. E. (2000). The labile nature of consolidation theory. *Nature Reviews Neuroscience,* 1, 216–219.

Nakamura, K., Dehaene, S., Jobert, A., Le Bihan, D. & Kouider, S. (2005). Subliminal convergence of Kanji and Kana words: Further evidence for functional parcellation of the posterior temporal cortex in visual word perception. *Journal of Cognitive Neuroscience,* 17, 954–968.

Nauta, W. J. (1971). The problem of the frontal lobe: A reinterpretation. *Journal of Psychiatric Research,* 8, 167–187.

Nisbett, R. E. & Wilson, T. D. (1977). Telling more than we can know: Verbal reports on mental processes. *Psychological Review,* 84, 231–259.

Nordbrandt, H. (2002). *Døden fra Lübeck.* København: Gyldendal.

O'Doherty, J., Kringelbach, M. L., Rolls, E. T., Hornak, J. & Andrews, C. (2001). Abstract reward and punishment representations in the human orbitofrontal cortex. *Nature Neuroscience,* 4, 95–102.

Ogawa, S., Lee, T. M., Kay, A. R. & Tank, D. W. (1990). Brain magnetic resonance imaging with contrast dependent on blood oxygenation. *Proceedings of the National Academy of Science United States of America,* 87, 9868–9872.

Olds, J. & Milner, P. (1954). Positive reinforcement produced by electrical stimulation of the septal area and other regions of rat brain. *Journal of Comparative and Physiological Psychology,* 47, 419–427.

Pakkenberg, B. (1990). Pronounced reduction of total neuron number in mediodorsal thalamic nucleus and nucleus accumbens in schizophrenics. *Archives of General Psychiatry,* 47, 1023–1028.

Pakkenberg, B. (1992). The volume of the mediodorsal thalamic nucleus in treated and untreated schizophrenics. *Schizophrenia Research,* 7, 95–100.

Pammer, K., Hansen, P. C., Kringelbach, M. L., Holliday, I. E., Barnes, G. R., Hillebrand, A., et al. (2004). Visual word recognition: The first half second. *Neuroimage,* 22, 1819–1825.

Panksepp, J. (1999). *Affective Neuroscience*. Oxford: Oxford University Press.

Pantev, C., Ross, B., Fujioka, T., Trainor, L. J., Schulte, M. & Schulz, M. (2003). Music and learning-induced cortical plasticity. *Annals of the New York Academy of Sciences*, 999, 438–450.

Papez, J. W. (1927). A proposed mechanism for emotion. *Archives of Neurology and Psychiatry*, 38, 725–743.

Payne, K. (1998). *Silent Thunder. In the Presence of Elephants*. London: Allan Lane Press.

Peciña, S. & Berridge, K. C. (2005). Hedonic hot spot in nucleus accumbens shell: Where do mu-opioids cause increased hedonic impact of sweetness? *The Journal of Neuroscience*, 25, 11777–11786.

Penfield, W. & Rasmussen, T. (1950). *The cerebral cortex of man: A clinical study of localization of function*. New York, NY: Macmillan.

Petrovic, P. & Ingvar, M. (2002). Imaging cognitive modulation of pain processing. *Pain*, 95, 1–5.

Petrovic, P., Kalso, E., Petersson, K. M. & Ingvar, M. (2002). Placebo and opioid analgesia—imaging a shared neuronal network. *Science*, 295, 1737–1740.

Phelps, M. E., Hoffman, E. J., Mullani, N. A. & Ter-Pogossian, M. M. (1975). Application of annihilation coincidence detection to transaxial reconstruction tomography. *Journal of Nuclear Medicine*, 16, 210–224.

Posner, M. & Raichle, M. E. (1997). *Images of Mind 2nd ed*. New York, NY: W H Freeman.

Price, C. J. & Devlin, J. T. (2003). The myth of the visual word form area. *Neuroimage*, 19, 473–481.

Proust, M. (1914). *À La Recherche Du Temps Perdu*. Paris: Gallimard.

Pulsifer, M. B., Brandt, J., Salorio, C. F., Vining, E. P., Carson, B. S. & Freeman, J. M. (2004). The cognitive outcome of hemispherectomy in 71 children. *Epilepsia*, 45, 243–254.

Purcell, E. M., Torry, H. C. & Pound, R. V. (1946). Resonance absorption by nuclear magnetic moments in a solid. *Physiological Reviews*, 69, 37.

Raichle, M. E., MacLeod, A. M., Snyder, A. Z., Powers, W. J., Gusnard, D. A. & Shulman, G. L. (2001). A default mode of brain function. *Proceedings of the National Academy of Sciences of the United States of America*, 98, 676–682.

Ramachandran, V. S. & Hirstein, W. (1998). The perception of phantom limbs. The D. O. Hebb lecture. *Brain*, 121 (Pt 9), 1603–1630.

Ramachandran, V. S. & Hubbard, E. M. (2003). Hearing colors, tasting shapes. *Scientific American*, 288, 52–59.

Ramachandran, V. S. & Rogers-Ramachandran, D. (1996). Synaesthesia in phantom limbs induced with mirrors. *Proceedings of the Royal Society of London. Series B, Containing papers of a biological character. Royal Society (Great Britain)*, 263, 377–386.

Ramachandran, V. S. & Rogers-Ramachandran, D. (2000). Phantom limbs and neural plasticity. *Archives of neurology*, 57, 317–320.

Redouté, J., Stoléru, S., Grégoire, M. C., Costes, N., Cinotti, L., Lavenne, F., et al. (2000). Brain processing of visual sexual stimuli in human males. *Human Brain Mapping*, 11, 162–177.

Rizzolatti, G., Camarda, R., Fogassi, L., Gentilucci, M., Luppino, G. & Matelli, M. (1988). Functional organization of inferior area 6 in the macaque monkey. II. Area F5 and the control of distal movements. *Experimental brain research. Experimentelle Hirnforschung. Experimentation cerebrale*, 71, 491–507.

Rolls, B. J., Rolls, E. T., Rowe, E. A. & Sweeney, K. (1981). Sensory specific satiety in man. *Physiology and Behavior*, 27, 137–142.

Rolls, E. T. (1999). *The Brain and Emotion*. Oxford: Oxford University Press.

Rolls, E. T., Inoue, K. & Browning, A. (2003). Activity of primate subgenual cingulate cortex neurons is related to sleep. *Journal of Neurophysiology*, 90, 134–142.

Rozin, P. (2001). Food Preference. In N. J. Smelser & P. B. Baltes (Eds.), *International Encyclopedia of the Social & Behavioral Sciences* (pp. 5719–5722). Amsterdam: Elsevier.

Rumelhart, D. E., Hinton, G. E. & Williams, R. J. (1986). Learning internal representations by error propagation. In D. E. Rumelhart & J. L. McClelland (Eds.), *Parallel Distributed*

Processing: Explorations in the Microstructure of Cognition (*Vol. 1*, pp. 318–364). Cambridge, MA: MIT Press.

Sacks, O. W. (1985). *The Man Who Mistook His Wife for a Hat*. London: Duckworth.

Salmelin, R., Hansen, P. C. & Kringelbach, M. L. (2007). *MEG. An Introduction to Methods*. New York, NY: Oxford University Press.

Savage-Rumbaugh, S. & Lewin, R. (1994). *Kanzi: The Ape at the Brink of the Human Mind*. New York, NY: Wiley.

Schacter, D. (1999). *Searching For Memory. The Brain, the Mind and the past*. New York, NY: Basic Books.

Scherz, G. (1968). Steno and brain research in the seventeenth century: Proceedings of the International Historical Symposium on Nicolaus Steno and brain research in the seventeenth century held in Copenhagen, 18–20 August, 1965, [1st] edn. Pergamon: Oxford.

Schnider, A. (2003). Spontaneous confabulation and the adaptation of thought to ongoing reality. *Nature Reviews Neuroscience*, 4, 662–671.

Schroeder, T. (2004). *Three Faces of Desire*. Oxford: Oxford University Press.

Schultz, W. W., van Andel, P., Sabelis, I. & Mooyaart, E. (1999). Magnetic resonance imaging of male and female genitals during coitus and female sexual arousal. BMJ, 319, 1596–1600.

Schwarz, E. (1929). Das Vorkommen des Schimpansen auf den linken Kongo-Ufer. *Revue de zoologie et de botanique africaines*, 16, 425–426.

Shaywitz, B. A., Shaywitz, S. E., Blachman, B. A., Pugh, K. R., Fulbright, R. K., Skudlarski, P., et al. (2004). Development of left occipitotemporal systems for skilled reading in children after a phonologically—based intervention. *Biological Psychiatry*, 55, 926–933.

Sherrington, C. S. (1951). *Man On His Nature*. Cambridge: Cambridge University Press.

Simon, O., Mangin, J. F., Cohen, L., Le Bihan, D. & Dehaene, S. (2002). Topographical layout of hand, eye, calculation, and language-related areas in the human parietal lobe. *Neuron*, 33, 475–487.

Skinner, B. F. (1938). *The Behavior of Organisms: An Experimental Analysis*. New York, NY: Appleton-Century.

Sokoloff, L., Reivich, M., Kennedy, C., Des Rosiers, M. H., Patlak, C. S., Pettigrew, K. D., Sakurada, O. & Shinohara, M. (1977). The [14C]deoxyglucose method for the measurement of local cerebral glucose utilization: Theory, procedure, and normal values in the conscious and anesthetized albino rat. *Journal of Neurochemistry*, 28, 897–916.

Sommer, M., Koch, M. A., Paulus, W., Weiller, C. & Buchel, C. (2002). Disconnection of speech-relevant brain areas in persistent developmental stuttering. *Lancet*, 360, 380–383.

Sperry, R. W. (1961). Cerebral organization and behavior. *Science*, 133, 1749–1757.

Squire, L. R. & Kandel, E. R. (1999). *Memory: From Mind to Molecules*. New York, NY: W.H. Freeman & Co.

Steinbeck, J. & Ricketts, E. F. (1941). *The Log from the Sea of Cortez*. London: Penguin.

Steinbuch, K. (1961). Die lernmatrix. *Kybernetik*, 1, 36–45.

Steno, N. (1950). *A Dissertation on the Anatomy of the Brain: Read in the Assembly Held in M. Thévenot's House in the Year 1665*. København: Nyt Nordisk Forlag.

Stern, K. & McClintock, M. K. (1998). Regulation of ovulation by human pheromones. *Nature*, 392, 177–179.

Sutherland, S. (1992). *Irrationality. The Enemy within*. London: Constable and Co.

Sutton, J. (2001). Descartes, René. In: *Encyclopedia of Life Sciences. Chichester: Wiley. http://www.els.net [doi:10.1038/npg.els.0002472]*.

Swanson, L. W. & Petrovich, G. D. (1998). What is the amygdala? *Trends in Neurosciences*, 21, 323–331.

Tarkiainen, A., Helenius, P., Hansen, P. C., Cornelissen, P. L. & Salmelin, R. (1999). Dynamics of letter string perception in the human occipitotemporal cortex. *Brain*, 122 (Pt 11), 2119–2132.

Ter-Pogossian, M. M., Phelps, M. E., Hoffman, E. J. & Mullani, N. A. (1975). A positron-emission transaxial tomograph for nuclear imaging (PETT). *Radiology*, 114, 89–98.

Thorndike, E. L. (1911). *Animal Intelligence: Experimental Studies.* New York, NY: Macmillan.

Thornhill-Miller, B. (2007). Creativity, religion, and the extraordinary-ordinary theory of novelty and the numinous. In D. Wulff (Ed.), *Handbook on the Psychology of Religion.* Oxford: Oxford University Press.

Tiihonen, J., Kuikka, J., Kupila, J., Partanen, K., Vainio, P., Airaksinen, J., et al. (1994). Increase in cerebral blood flow of right prefrontal cortex in man during orgasm. *Neuroscience Letters,* 170, 241–243.

Tratz, E. P. & Heck, H. (1954). Der afrikanische Anthropoide "Bonobo": Eine neue Menschenaffengattung. *Säugertierkundliche Mitteilungen,* 2, 97–101.

Tsao, D. Y., Freiwald, W. A., Tootell, R. B. & Livingstone, M. S. (2006). A cortical region consisting entirely of face-selective cells. *Science,* 311, 670–674.

Turing, A. (1950). Computing machinery and intelligence. *Mind,* 59, 433–460.

Völlm, B. A., de Araujo, I. E. T., Cowen, P. J., Rolls, E. T., Kringelbach, M. L., Smith, K. A., et al. (2004). Methamphetamine activates reward circuitry in drug naïve human subjects. *Neuropsychopharmacology,* 29, 1715–1722.

Vrba, J. & Robinson, S. E. (2001). Signal processing in magnetoencephalography. *Methods,* 25, 249–271.

Wagner, A. D., Bunge, S. A. & Badre, D. (2004). Cognitive control, semantic memory, and priming: Contributions from prefrontal cortex. In M. S. Gazzaniga (Ed.), *The Cognitive Neurosciences 3rd ed.* Cambridge, MA: MIT Press.

Walsh, V. & Pascual-Leone, A. (2003). *Transcranial Magnetic Stimulation. A Neurochronometrics of Mind.* Cambridge, MA: MIT Press.

Warrington, E. K. & Shallice, T. (1980). Word-form dyslexia. *Brain,* 103, 99–112.

Wedekind, C., Seebeck, T., Bettens, F. & Paepke, A. (1995). MHC-dependent mate preferences in humans. *Proceedings of the Royal Society of London. Series B, Containing papers of a Biological character. Royal Society (Great Britain),* 260, 245–249.

Wegner, D. M. (2002). *The Illusion of Conscious Will.* Cambridge, MA: MIT Press.

Weiskrantz, L. (1997). *Consciousness Lost and Found.* Oxford: Oxford University Press.

Weiskrantz, L., Elliott, J. & Darlington, C. (1971). Preliminary observations on tickling oneself. *Nature,* 230, 598–599.

Wernicke, C. (1874). *Der aphasische Symptomencomplex. Eine psychologische Studie auf anatomischer Basis*: Breslau: Cohn and Weigert.

Wilson, E. O. (1975). *Sociobiology: The New Synthesis.* Cambridge, MA: Belknap Press.

Wilson, E. O. (1995). *Naturalist.* New York, NY: Warner Books.

Wilson, E. O. (1998). *Consilience: The Unity of Knowledge.* New York, NY: Knopf.

Wilson, T. D. (2002). *Strangers to Ourselves: Discovering the Adaptive Unconscious.* Cambridge, MA: Harvard University Press.

Winchester, S. (1999). *The Surgeon of Crowthorne: A Tale of Murder, Madness and the Oxford English Dictionary.* Oxford: Oxford University Press.

Winchester, S. (2003). *The meaning of everything: The story of the Oxford English Dictionary.* Oxford: Oxford University Press.

Winkielman, P., Berridge, K. C. & Wilbarger, J. L. (2005). Unconscious affective reactions to masked happy versus angry faces influence consumption behavior and judgments of value. *Personality and social psychology bulletin,* 31, 121–135.

Wolpert, L. (2000). *Malignant Sadness: The Anatomy of Depression.* London: Free Press.

Wrangham, R. W., McGrew, W. C., de Waal, F. B. M. & Heltne, P. G. (1994). *Chimpanzee cultures.* Cambridge, MA: Harvard University Press.

Yarbus, A. L. (1967). *Eye movements and Vision.* New York, NY: Plenum Press.

Zeki, S. (1993). *A vision of the Brain.* Oxford: Blackwell scientific.

Zumpe, D. & Michael, R. P. (1968). The clutching reaction and orgasm in the female rhesus monkey (Macaca mulatta). *The Journal of Endocrinology,* 40, 117–123.

ACKNOWLEDGMENTS

Writing this book was a great pleasure which was not as solitary as one might imagine. The ideas in this book were shaped not in solitude but with those friends that make life worth living. Foremost my greatest debt is to my editor Catharine Carlin who gave me advice at every stage of the project and whom together with Steve Holtje, Nicholas Liu, and Ronnie Lipton greatly improved the final manuscript with their detailed and penetrating comments.

I am grateful to those who shared their great expertise with me, on a variety of topics, over the years: Kent Berridge whose contributions to the science of pleasure are unparalleled; and to Bent Foltmann, Rodney Michael John Cotterill, and Stanislas Dehaene for their penetrating insights into the nature of evolutionary brain function. In Oxford I have, over the years, had the very good fortune to learn from some brilliant scientists: Susan Iversen, Alan Stein, and Tipu Aziz. At the *The Queen's College*, Oxford, it has been a joy to share many discussions with Sir Alan Budd, Samantha Besson, Alex Green, Peter McLeod, Peter Neumann, Chris

Norbury, Jim Reed, Peter Robbins, Maria Schonbek, Jackie Stedall and my other dear colleagues. In Aarhus, I thank my colleagues: Ole Fejerskov, Albert Gjedde, Hans Lou, Arne Møller, Andreas Roepstorff, Henriette Vuust, Peter Vuust, and Leif Østergaard.

The scientists whose insights have helped shape some of the ideas in this book include: Jean-Pierre Changeux, Piers Cornelissen, Phil Cowen, Tom Cullen, Antonio Damasio, Richard Davidson, Martin Davies, Ivan De Araujo, Nico Frijda, John Geake, Guy Goodwin, Jeffrey Gray, Richard Gregory, Peter Hansen, Paul Harris, Peter Hobden, Jan Kalbitzer, Joseph Ledoux, Siri Leknes, Paul Matthews, John O'Doherty, Sarah Owen, Jaak Panksepp, Predrag Petrovic, Robert Rogers, Matthew Rushworth, Branden Thornhill-Miller, and Larry Weiskrantz. In addition, I have been fortunate to work with the artist Annie Cattrell.

My research is generously funded by the TrygFonden Charitable Foundation. Parts of this book has also been supported by the Ulla and Mogens Folmer Andersen Foundation and Learning Lab, Denmark.

Good friends have contributed in many important ways: Trine Beckett, NanaKi Bonfils, David Bouchet, Janne Breinholt Bak, Claudia Canales, Maria Cannata, Joris Capenberghs, Mads Christoffersen, Tristan Cordier, Karim Dahou, Tarik Dahou, Antonia Duffy, Adam Engell, Vilhelm Engell, Robin Engelhardt, Inge Foltmann, Jérôme Gérard, Suzanne Giese, Nafy Guèye, Richard Hart, Colin Jennings, Mogens Klostergaard Jensen, Erna Kringelbach, Lis Larsen, Simon Mason, Dermot McNulty, Susanne Milne, Yann Nachtman, Karsten Nielsen, Kathryn Nwajiaku, Klaus

Petersen, Sølvi Sand, Aminatou Sar, Yandé Sène, Loredana Soceneantu, Hélène Sow, David Stavnstrup, Jakob Stavnstrup, Peter Stenbæk, George Stroup, Christian Teller, Janne Teller, Virginie Vanhaeverbeke, and Vibe Wilkens.

The support of my family has mattered more to me than they will ever know: my parents Gregers and Birgit Kringelbach and my sister Louise Kringelbach. Most of all, I thank my wife Hélène Neveu Kringelbach and our daughters Maya and Laura for making peace, love, and understanding.

INDEX

(References to figures are in *italics*)

D